# FIBROMYALGIA
## Well-Being

DEE CAMPBELL

BALBOA.
PRESS

A DIVISION OF HAY HOUSE

Cover Design Concept: Chenoa Raggatt

Balboa Press books may be ordered through booksellers or by contacting:

Balboa Press
A Division of Hay House
1663 Liberty Drive
Bloomington, IN 47403
www.balboapress.com.au
1-(877) 407-4847

ISBN: 978-1-4525-0536-7 (sc)
ISBN: 978-1-4525-0537-4 (e)

Printed in the United States of America

Balboa Press rev. date: 06/05/2012

# DEDICATION

To my beautiful daughter Chenoa and wonderful
partner Brenton, who have always encouraged
and believed in ME.

# CONTENTS

Foreword ....................................................................... ix

Acknowledgements...................................................... xi

Introduction............................................................... xiii

## PART ONE

Insights into my life—the first 30 years ................... 3

Subtle illness (2000-2007) .......................................... 21

The 'Crash' That Led To Diagnosis........................ 34

Important Decisions In 2011.................................... 53

## PART TWO

My Team Of Health Professionals .......................... 65

Resources And Strategies....................................... 100

Do your best, Rest (sleep) Repeat ........................ 147

It takes both rain and sunshine For a
beautiful rainbow to appear!................................... 159

Looking Ahead—The Four Of Us....................... 174

Destination Unknown!............................................ 183

Afterword................................................................. 191

Appendix One ............................................................ 201
    Dr Teitelbaums article 'From Fatigued to
    Fantastic! You Can Effectively treat CFS,
    Fatigue, Fibromyalgia, ME and Muscle
    Pain' (used with permission, 2012).
Appendix Two ............................................................ 212
    Positive And Useful Quotes To Ponder
Appendix Three ......................................................... 220
    Useful Resources List
Appendix Four .......................................................... 230
    Recommended Books

# Foreword

A holistic approach to wellbeing suggests that wellness occurs when the many domains of human functioning are nurtured; and when individuals are connected to self, to others and to the world.

Approaches that target the various areas of a person's life are most likely to be successful in terms of bringing lasting growth and positive change.

In this book, Dee draws upon significant personal experience to provide readers with a very real and tangible application of these approaches.

Tracey Jane

Clinical Psychologist.

# Acknowledgements

I wish to acknowledge Stephen Hadges, my wonderful GP for his ongoing support, dedicated approach and understanding. His willingness to work WITH me (over the last 5 years) has greatly assisted the process and empowered me. Also; to Maureen Thomson (my Naturopath), for adding more depth and an additional (much needed) perspective to my journey. Thanks also to Tracey Jane (clinical psychologist) who provided another vital element and shared her profound knowledge and valuable resources with me. I also acknowledge the many 'Complementary Health Practitioners' who have assisted me in obtaining a richer understanding of myself and the direct relationships between physical health and our Emotional and Spiritual wellbeing.

I also Thank Jacob Teitelbaum, MD; for his specialised expertise and contribution in this area, as well as his ongoing commitment to enhance the lives of people with fibromyalgia and chronic fatigue syndrome (and related health issues)—all around the world.

Information has been included from the book *'From Fatigued to Fantastic'* by Jacob Teitelbaum, M.D: 2007,

Penguin Group, New York (including references to SHINE protocol), and has been used with permission.

I also offer my deepest gratitude to the network of people that have supported and encouraged me through the process of writing this book, especially close friends, contributors (sponsors), Tania Hayes (Author of 'Love Has No Limits'; 2008) and the dear Eugene (Gene) McClarty. Gene wrote a book entitled 'Live Life to The Full', in 2006 at the age of 89 years 'young'. I drew from this book time and time again through challenging times, and based areas of this book upon his wisdom.

Gene is truly guiding testament to a life well lived! (Gene also kindly provided me with permission to draw inspiration from his book, and reproduce some of his work.)

My heartfelt gratitude is extended to all the individuals that have contributed and travelled this journey with me. Thank YOU for making my world, and therefore, OUR world a much better place.

# Introduction

The decision to write this book came from my own personal journey—as many books do. The most prominent deciding factor came from my desire to help others by sharing my own story. When I was struggling with this condition and the many elements of Fibromyalgia Syndrome (FMS)—I searched for explanations, books, evidence, resolutions, stories and the experiences of others that travelled this road before me. Endless searches provided me with some useful books and literature.

However I discovered that the information was mostly clinically based, and the personal stories I sought were scarce and highly needed. Whilst not many people close to me, really knew the depth and impacts (sometimes despair) of this condition, a few that *were* aware—and had known me for a long time—made suggestions now and then that perhaps I should write my own book—*'someday'*. However, it was not my intention until recently. Quite unusually, I had written notes, kept records and journalled thoughts along the way—and this proved very useful, when re-enacting the last 10 years!

My second reason for my decision to write this book was for the benefit of my family. You see, when one goes through this FMS journey—it is not just the person with the condition that travels. It is the people closest to you who travel along with you—and who are affected by the many elements and far reaching consequences. My partner and our daughter have been affected by this condition. I hope they may read this and gain perspective of how it's been for me, and this will shape their 'reality'. To obtain a better understanding of my behaviours, struggles, moods and actions—both good and bad—that may have been triggered or influenced by this condition. Our daughter is now aged 11 years, and she is old enough to grasp an understanding and deserves to have the opportunity to be a part of this reflective process, as it has affected her, and no doubt will continue to influence and shape her in the future.

My third reason was for myself. I hope that this process will provide some reflection and healing. That through this process I may even make some peace with my 'reality'.

I make some assumptions with this book. Most importantly the audience targeted are others dealing with this condition, their carers & families/friends and Professionals interested in the wellbeing of their patients. I make the presumption that a basic knowledge and understanding of **Fibromyalgia Syndrome** (FMS) is held by the reader. It is my story, and not a clinically written account that guides treatment plans etc. Although scarce, there are a few good resources around that discuss treatment options, research and also encapsulate lifestyle and holistic health. I wanted my contribution to be easy to read (people with FMS struggle to read for long periods), fairly brief and to the point and easy to connect with. I will leave the mechanics and the clinical aspects (and research) to those who are better qualified in this regard.

FMS is an extremely complex condition (thus the word 'syndrome'), with many complicated factors involved. My intention is to focus on MY story.

This book represents a personal account of what happened in my case—the impacts, the effects, my own pathways of treatment, and what was useful. I hope that some other people with this (FMS) and related condition(s) and readers will be able to 'connect' and get some reassurance for their own long term wellbeing.

That is not to say I recommend or suggest that anyone follow the same path, as we are all different and unique people who will be affected in different ways. We must all make our own decisions based on our own lifestyles, values etc—and take personal responsibility for those decisions, as best we can. What has worked for me may not work for you.

For me, I get great comfort from believing that I am grateful that one of my challenges in life has been FMS. You see, I believe no one is 'immune' to the suffering that life brings. At some time, we will all be faced with illness and/or disability, sadness and grief. However, FMS is not necessarily a life threatening illness. It is a great challenge and indeed a difficult journey—and most of the time, *overwhelming*. However, we need to keep this in perspective. Many people around us are afflicted with life threatening illness or situations that they too don't deserve. As most of you, I have known people undergoing the reality of chemotherapy and other similar treatments. I have known people to lose battles with brain tumours, cancer, to become disabled, and to become very ill. Many people around them also walk alongside them.

FMS has been very inconvenient, and not a very positive experience, however, I have been 'forced' to learn how to better manage my health and wellbeing. I have thus far been able to maintain my independence and I have still been able to enjoy some quality of life. It is my every intention to be blessed with the opportunity to watch my daughter grow into a woman, and enjoy all that brings—within some capacity. So, to me FMS is a challenge that I can hold some power.

Do I worry about my daughter suffering with this condition? It crosses my mind, but I don't dwell on it. If she does, we know we can try to navigate and manage it. Just because I have struggled with it doesn't necessarily mean that she will. She will have access to more tools that can assist her, if and when she needs them. We are also learning through this process and therefore, she may be better equipped to minimise some of the 'risk factors'.

Many people with cancer and other afflictions (including disabilities and special needs) don't 'deserve' their challenges and many would not have expected their illness/issues. They may have lived 'model lives' and done everything right—and still end up sick (or disabled). In our (FMS) case, we may be pre disposed to some risk factors of FMS (eg premature ovarian failure, thyroid problems etc) but it is that pre disposition **combined with** lifestyle and environmental influences that will determine the onset.

We don't necessarily choose our illness but somehow, when we are confronted with challenges, we need to accept the reality and continue to move forward—even if in baby steps.

My biggest suggestion to people who are travelling with FMS—***simplify, simplify, simplify!*** Life is hard enough and stressful enough without FMS. With FMS your capacity to cope with the same level of 'life' as you may have *pre FMS* days will be significantly diminished.

My other piece of advice would be to work really hard at understanding the difference between *physical* WELLNESS and WELL BEING.

They are quite different concepts and in my opinion— this will be the key to how well you manage and cope with long term management of FMS.

Although our wellbeing is greatly influenced by our state of physical wellness, the extent of negative influence is largely our own choice. We can still work towards a reasonably positive state of wellbeing, even amidst *physical* UNwellness.

Alternatively, I encourage everyone to begin to use a broader definition of **wellness** that includes physical, emotional (psychological) and spiritual aspects. This may be your greatest challenge!

I hope you get some comfort and connection from my experience(s). I begin with a little of my life history, 'pre FMS' life (subtle sickness), followed by days of diagnosis and treatment, leading to long term management. I share what I have tried, and I hope that you can become **well enough** *in the physical sense*, whilst also aiming for a state of **wellbeing** that provides you with an improved 'Mind-Body Connection', and therefore an enhanced quality of life. I hope you find it realistic, but most importantly I hope you find it helpful!

I always knew that I was a strong person. I have always tried to be proud of who I am and what I have achieved, albeit (like most of us) at times in very trying circumstances. However, FMS has truly taught me that I am now of STRONG CHARACTER . . . and I hope you *learn about yourself* as well, through this book and through your own experiences and journey with Fibromyalgia Syndrome.

# PART ONE

## CHAPTER ONE

# INSIGHTS INTO MY LIFE— THE FIRST 30 YEARS

As a child I was fairly quiet (shy), easy to get along with, easily made friends and coped with change due to being privy to many, varied childhood experiences. According to my *'School Leaver Statement'* in 1983 (before completing Year 11 High School; at the age of 15 years and 8 months)—

*'Dee is a pleasant, well groomed and exceptionally cooperative student who has made every effort to succeed. She is conscientious and reliable and may be depended upon to work to the best of her ability with a minimum of supervision. Dee is well liked and respected. She is friendly and supportive'.*

Through various networks, in younger (teenage) years, I have been described as—sensitive, reliable, industrious, cheerful, honest, refined and sensitive to the wellbeing of others, Professional thinker, efficient, friendly, likeable, sociable, helpful and polite. I like to think these traits are still travelling with me!

I have no recollection of being rebellious and recall a desire to work with children (child care) or with People with Disabilities.

At the age of 15 years, I joined the finance sector and remained in a major bank for 10 years exactly. Socially, the 'bank' lifestyle was busy, fun and very fulfilling. Life was always about planning our next night out, our next 'adventure', holiday, social activity, party etc. Mostly life circumstance dictated in many ways, as it does for many—as job security, full time employment, earning an income and setting oneself up for the future are all important.

When I was 25 years old and approaching 10 years' service—an opportunity presented to leave not only the security of employment, but also to leave Australian shores—to relocate to New Zealand. This was a welcome opportunity and very timely due to certain (stressful) challenges and experiences. All of which greatly influenced my decision for this move. It was a HUGE change, but I was excited about new beginnings.

In the time leading up to this change, life had delivered many highs and many, many lows. Decisions had been made with both positive and negative outcomes.

In hindsight, I guess I was searching for a 'purpose' and trying to make my own way in the world. Maybe, it could be said that I chose an 'escape route' with the hope for better outcomes and a fresh start. On another level, it was an opportunity to follow through a new career path and direction.

As it turned out, initial adaptation to the new surroundings proved difficult—and necessity prevailed again. Casual work, manual labour and multiple jobs were needed to make it through. I took on more seasonal work, and one job led into the next as result of my sound reputation and work ethic. For a while I was working day shift, night shift and fell into the next job and the 'slow down' never seemed to come. But, money was needed—to ensure I could eat, keep a roof over my head and survive.

Once I had become a little familiar with my new community and location I followed up on volunteering within this community—for an organisation that provided support services to People With Disabilities ('IHC'—'The New Zealand Society for the Intellectually Handicapped', a New Zealand Service Provider for People with Disabilities).

From there I juggled this volunteering with the seasonal (casual) employment, until I was able to move into paid employment with 'IHC'—beginning on a casual basis and then more permanent (contract) roles. I loved this area of work and undertook every work role and every presenting opportunity with passion and drive. At this same time, I began to discover a thirst for study and further education and learning. Perhaps this was partly due to leaving High School at a young age, or indeed fuelled by my belief that we are always learning and my openness and willingness to remain open to learning.

Life in New Zealand was busy, but after 3 years there I had the realisation that the time was right for me to return home to South Australia. Again, many factors influenced the dramatic change to return here. One thing was for sure, and that was my desire to continue on this newly found career path.

On one level, I had achieved one of the things I had set out to achieve and could now continue to build on this. I was Thankful that I had embarked on that part of my journey, I had given it my best—and on many levels, had made it!

I remained in the field of Disability Support for the following 6 years, and also continued to quench my thirst for learning and started a University Degree in Adelaide at the age of 30 years! Again, through most of this time (at University) necessity meant that study and work needed to be undertaken at the same time.

In every job I have had along the way, I've had a very good reputation. A strong work ethic also ensured life was busy but most importantly, that I was employed and earning a much needed income—which was crucial as I often had limited support around me.

From High School days I had a desire to work either as a teacher or to help others who are vulnerable and less fortunate than myself (eg People With Disabilities). This was underpinned by a passionate interest in 'community' and society. Consequently, alongside paid work (from a very young age) I also participated in voluntary work—and still continue to do so.

Throughout my 20's, life threw many challenges my way and sometimes my choices landed me in difficulty—but, I continued to search for that 'pot of gold'. Often I operated from survival mode and relied on adrenaline. Although some of my choices possibly added to my own challenges, they were always well intentioned at the time. It possibly looked to outsiders like I was undertaking a 'race', and my efforts were my attempt to get 'there' quicker.

Upon reflection I realise that in a 7 year timeframe (1991-1998)—I moved 'place of residence' approximately 11 times! Amongst these moves were many other added stressors (significant life experiences) and changes (location, employment, friends, support network, relationships etc). I'm not unique in this regard and in no way do I seek a 'pity party' or sympathy.

Fight-flight mode often got me through and kept me going—albeit not **consciously**—but deep down I guess I always hoped and believed that I would find happiness, fulfilment and MYSELF. I had a desire to find out who I was and what made me tick, and I have always needed to do this IN MY OWN WAY. I think we all strive for this, and I certainly am still on this path BUT I can say that I am more aware now than I ever have been. The best way to achieve these wonderful things called contentment and fulfilment is to try to have a **conscious awareness** in all that we do.

Along this journey I've had some amazing and brilliant people come across my path. Some stayed only briefly and some are still involved in this journey and are still walking with me—as I no longer run. BUT, they have all made imprints on my heart and I value each and every one of them for the impact they have made on the person I have now become.

## Deidre meets Brenton (1998)

Brenton and I as individuals had no intention to meet up, and life was certainly busy for both of us at the time we met. As they say, you usually end up finding love when you least expect it—or when you have given up on looking for it! This was certainly true for me, due to my previous outcomes with relationships.

Life was ticking along and finally I felt like I was moving in the right direction—although still struggling through. And then Brenton and I crossed paths. Initially we intended to take our relationship slowly, as we both really needed to be sure. By nature we are both very cautious people (some may say 'stubborn'!) and both born under horoscope star sign of Capricorn. However, it all fell into place—at a reasonably rapid pace. We have no regrets from that!

From the first time we met, we felt like we had known each other forever. There was so many feelings of 'meant to be together'. I felt like the stars had been aligned that night and am extremely grateful Brenton crossed my path. The timing was perfect, and we were where we 'were meant to be'.

It felt so 'right', like I had met him and known him before. I had not experienced that upon meeting anyone else in my 30 years. It was indeed like 'finding my other half'.

We had different interests and were dis similar in regards to taste in music, food and some other things. On the other hand our values, behaviours, and spiritual beliefs were aligned. I have always been able to talk to Brenton and express myself—without feeling judged or ridiculed. Although he is more private than me—there are lots of 'knowing ness' es.

Even now, 14 years on, we will often think the same thoughts and buy the same thing and come home with something very similar. Sometimes this is handy, sometimes it's freaky. We do have different thoughts about some things but I think this is healthy. But, our foundations seem to be the same. We have a very solid and firm foundation and it's always felt quite unshakable!!

What I immediately loved about Brenton was his calmness, kindness and gentleness. I admired his sensitivity and ability to pick up on things that others would have no interest in. I knew immediately that I wanted to share more time with him and build on something that was very peaceful and solid. When we were together I never wanted to return to reality. When we were together everything just fell into place.

Brenton never questioned me about my past and never judged me for that. That in itself meant a lot to me, as I feel like he knew me for who I was.

It was like he knew and loved the REAL Deidre, rather than the one presenting. In some ways upon reflection, I think he knew ME better than I knew MYSELF. It was simple and flowed, like a beautiful story. We made our own story and each of us provided the other with complementing characteristics. He was more reserved and private and I was open and friendly. I had lived in many different places and environments and moved around a lot, Brenton had only ever lived in one home and then his own place. On top of everything else—he was my solid, calming and grounding influence. We complemented and completed each other.

Although we have never married, we have always felt connected and very secure in our relationship. We may marry one day—but for now—we are both content and very happy within our family unit.

## CHANGE IN CAREER DIRECTION— CARERS (2001 ONWARDS)

Just over 8 years was spent in employment with People With Disabilities, both in New Zealand and here in Australia. I found this work very fulfilling and look back on that time with great admiration for the wonderful people I worked with—both service users and staff. These environments were great teachers of life and of love. I loved the opportunities I was given to enhance Quality of Life and opportunities for People with Disabilities, within the community. I had a passion and commitment to do whatever I could in this regard, as this work deserves nothing less! It was an honour and a privilege to contribute to making a positive difference.

Through this work, I often found myself working within home environments, and this introduced me to a new group of people—CARERS. These include family members, friends (and neighbours) who provide care and support to the most vulnerable members of our society—People with Disabilities (including special needs), people with chronic mental/ physical illness, and older people. A shift from Deinstitutionalisation to community care resulted in movements and changes within policy and this was the beginning of a career for me that valued (unpaid) carers. I had utmost respect and admiration for carers and was passionate about recognising carers and placing them in a more valued place within our society.

Often, the 'vulnerable' person was the focus of services and interventions and thus the carers were sometimes left feeling undervalued and unrecognised. So, I hoped that through further study (University degree) I would be able to make a positive and well deserving difference to the lives of carers and therefore to society. However, I stress that my contribution pales into significance—in comparison to what carers contribute to our community, economy and to society each and every day.

Earlier on, I moved into a role that focussed on systemic advocacy and this provided a firm foundation in regards to service delivery and in turn provided an understanding of the role, function and benefits of *Carer support*. I moved into *carer support* and felt confident that I had empathy, respect and the understanding needed to fulfil a role with direct contact with carers. I also felt that I had the capacity (through skills and knowledge base)—to influence change and further advocate, raise community awareness and thus enhance community acknowledgement of their role and the critical part they (Carers) play within society.

*Carer support* seeks to balance the scales—to refocus on the CARER. Hopefully, Carer support adds to individual resilience and supports the long term sustainability (and enhanced wellbeing) of the carer. Carers are always working behind the scenes, getting on with the many jobs and responsibilities they have. Through Carer support, I have been surrounded by people who demonstrate the true meaning of courage, strength, and resilience. Carers have many other qualities, but out of love and necessity they continue to face many challenges. Often not knowing what they will be confronted with next, around the next corner—but continually finding the strength and courage to go around the next corner anyway. They are amazing, remarkable people who have an amazing capacity to cope with stress and catastrophe whilst showing great determination to always do the very best that they can—for the person(s) they care for. They are truly the 'givers' of this world and bring a whole new perspective to the word LOVE.

Through building relationships with carers and being involved with the role of carer support, I have learned to appreciate and value life. I have seen how quickly life can change and developed a deep appreciation of how fragile life is; and I have worked alongside Carers who have shown such great quality of character.

*Carer support* offers mutual support, facilitates encouragement and caring, provides opportunities for participation, supports social networks, facilitates and nurtures linkages to other services and support (formal and informal), and thus aims to reduce or overcome social isolation throughout this process.

My role in carer support has been to initiate and facilitate a non-judgemental environment, predominantly via carer support groups and sessions. Ideally, this environment aims to offer— mutual support, shared experiences, friendship and acceptance. It's hoped that this environment enables carers to come together, feel supported and included, feel listened to, valued and appreciated. They may share stories, information, obtain guidance and strategies that further support the very important work that they do—with minimal (if any) financial payment and (often) with minimal acknowledgement or recognition from our society.

I have always undertaken this work with great passion and integrity—as it so deserves. My respect and admiration for the personal value of each individual carer, as well as the role they fulfil—make it a very meaningful profession. A profession that indeed gives me back so much more than I could ever contribute. It is interwoven in my own character and this theme and the importance of this career influence on me personally, will return later in the story.

# FIBROMYALGIA EXPLAINED

Fibromyalgia is often referred to as a 'chronic multi system illness' (CMI). It is sometimes defined as a musculo skeletal disorder' BUT in my opinion—it is so much more than this. With far reaching effects and symptoms, as I will now explain to the best of my ability.

The symptoms may include (but are NOT limited to)—

Stiffness, widespread pain (including achiness), unrelenting and overwhelming fatigue/extreme exhaustion, sleep disorders (unrefreshing sleep), hormonal dysfunction, increased allergies, brain/cognitive dysfunction (confusion and memory problems), anxiety and depression, frequent/recurrent infections and immune dysfunction, bowel dysfunction, weight gain, and a reduced ability to tolerate and manage stress. It is thought that these symptoms may occur as result of hypothalamus, pituitary and/or adrenal problems (possible 'underfunctioning').

**Dr Jacob Teitelbaum, MD** offers a more comprehensive explanation at the end of this book ('appendix one'), however, in a nutshell—

## 'What is causing these Illnesses? ...

*CFS, Fibromyalgia and MPS (Myofascial pain) are not a single illness. Our study has shown that they are a mix of many different processes that can be triggered by many causes. Some patients had their illness caused by any of a number of infections. In this situation, many people can identify the time that their illness began almost to the day. This is also the case in those patients who had an injury (sometimes very mild) that was strong enough to disrupt their sleep and trigger this process.*

*In others the illness had a more gradual onset. This may have been associated with hormonal deficiencies (eg low thyroid, estrogen, testosterone, cortisone etc) despite normal blood tests. In others, it may be associated with chronic stress, antibiotic use with secondary yeast overgrowth, and/or nutritional deficiencies. Indeed, we have found well over 100 common causes of, and factors that contribute to, these syndromes.*

*What these processes have in common is that most of them can suppress a major control centre in your brain called the hypothalamus. This centre controls sleep, your hormonal system, temperature and blood flow/pressure. When you don't sleep deeply, your immune system also stops working properly and you'll be in pain. When we realised this, the myriad symptoms seen in CFS and fibromyalgia suddenly made sense'.*

Fibromyalgia therefore, involves the whole body and potentially throws all kinds of things 'out of balance'.

Fibromyalgia can take someone who is educated, ambitious, hardworking and tireless AND rob them of their ability to work, clean the house, exercise, think clearly and ever feel awake OR healthy! However, it's NOT 'burn out', or depression, or laziness, or whingeing, or psychologically driven. It IS the result of widespread dysfunction in the body and the brain that is hard to understand, difficult to treat and thus far impossible to cure.

**From our perspective;**

It is indeed a complex condition that is difficult to understand, and it can impact on every part of the body. It can be confusing for others to understand, as symptoms may fluctuate and often people misinterpret the symptoms and decide fibromyalgia must be a psychological problem. However, more and more scientific evidence is proving that it is in fact a very real, physical condition.

People with fibromyalgia may not always appear sick (as they may with other chronic conditions). This is due to levels of hormones and other substances involved which may fluctuate, and rise and fall in response to different situations and conditions. The more a person may be 'out of the zone' then the worse they may feel.

(For this reason, it's hard for other people to 'see' when a person struggles with fatigue and other symptoms, and what's difficult to see, is indeed difficult to understand. Naturally enough, most people with FMS and related symptoms are housebound (restricted or absent socially etc.) whilst at their worst times and/or during flare up 'episodes'. So, most people only really see them when they are functional.)

The dysfunction in the person's body may turn mild pressure or even an itch into pain. Essentially the brain amplifies signals and 'turns up the volume' of everything. This can include light, noise and odour on top of pain and may result in further overloaded system(s). These factors also cause additional 'stress' on the body, of which the body cannot cope with effectively.

Stress and stressful situations may also make symptoms worse. We all respond to physical and emotional stress, hormones kick in and the body adapts and usually deals with what it's confronted with. However, people with fibromyalgia may have trouble physically regulating these hormones and this makes stress difficult and may trigger symptoms. Stress in this context includes emotional stress and also physical stress—including illness, lack of sleep, nutritional deficiencies, infections and injuries.

The fatigue of fibromyalgia is not just tiredness BUT utter exhaustion. In comparison to a person who may have stayed up all night studying, or up feeding a baby, or caring for a sick child, or perhaps experiencing the flu. If you take any of these situations and consider on top of this self-care, taking care of work, raising children, cleaning the house, preparing meals and continued functioning.

In most of these cases a few good sleeps would alleviate this tired and exhausted feeling. However, this is often constant and ongoing for people with fibromyalgia, and further complicated by accompanying sleep disorders (often together with pain) that make a good night's sleep a rare and precious gift! These sleep issues then may also further exacerbate hormonal deficiencies thus resulting in further dysfunction at physical systemic level.

(With fibromyalgia comes sleep disorders that make a good night's sleep a rarity. A person with fibromyalgia will most likely encounter sleep disorders and ongoing issues with sleep maintenance.

Of course, sleep is crucial for restoration of the body (cells, hormones, muscles etc) which in turn renews the body's energy systems. Sleep issues and deprivation on the other hand—cause many implications—many of which are grossly underestimated by most people!)

CHAPTER TWO

# SUBTLE ILLNESS (2000-2007)

It is stated time and time again in books and documentation and research about FMS that most people that are diagnosed with the condition have been 'typically Type A Over achievers'. Of course, this aspect will be a saving grace when in the midst of despair (as this part of our personality stops us from crumbling) BUT the reality check is that it is also likely to be part of the cause of the initial problem as well.

Throw into this mix a few pre disposed elements that also affect the energy systems (thyroid, pituitary)—then you have a recipe for potential disaster.

As most of you may now understand, FMS is your body's way of coping with an 'overloaded' system. If we have one or two under functioning elements within our energy system, then this puts more stress and pressure on to the next, and so on—until all those systems that create our energy (and have other important functions) actually can't cope anymore, crash and thus the body operates in an under functioning state.

If these systems all crash together = FMS. So now I have a bit of understanding of how my lifestyle may have contributed to high levels of stress for my physical body—along with some physical predisposed 'weaknesses' and environmental influences, and I never once gave any of this any thought!

Up until my early 30's I had never suffered or endured much illness. Never needed to take sick days or time off, rarely even had the need for medicine—even Paracetamol. My health had never caused me concern and I rarely saw Doctors. In fact, I didn't even have a regular Doctor.

Brenton and I met in 1998, when I was aged 30 years. I was studying for my University degree (Bachelor of Social Science—Human Services), doing voluntary work and also undertaking paid work at the time.

For some reason, approx. 18 months into our relationship I had a GP visit, and discovered at that time I had 'hormonal imbalance'. In fact, I was informed by this GP that 'if I intended to have children, then I would be wise not to leave this too late'.

This GP was of the opinion that it was highly likely I would experience early menopause. This jolted me to the core!

It was also around this time I began to experience headaches but avoided taking any medications—as I found I was very sensitive to many medicines. To the extent that often the side effects would be far worse than the symptom!

There are a couple of other significant points worth mentioning here—as looking back I can see their relationship with what was later to develop.

Weight management had never been easy for me. Although I thought my diet was 'reasonable' and didn't over eat or eat fatty, creamy or bad junk foods—my weight was never easy to keep within 'healthy range'. This continued to be source of aggravation and got worse in the following years. This is still something that I struggle with to this day.

My loathing of shopping and shopping centres was another interesting phenomenon. The bright lighting and my sensitivity to the environment has gotten worse over the years.

After a short time, I need to get out and back into fresh air. The lights, the sounds, smells etc make me feel quite light headed and 'spaced out'—like I am dreaming. I become *ultra-sensitive* to absolutely everything that one encounters whilst there.

Within this environment I also get a headache, and get very cranky! And thus, this takes away any enjoyment from these experiences. This is something I remember from around 8 to 10 years ago, and can still only tolerate short episodes and avoid it at all, if I can! If I bump into people I know—they must think I am very vague or very weird, as I am just such a different person in this environment and I am aware of the changes to my personality! (Over the years this has become increasingly significant with shops and also other venues where lighting, sounds and smell are factors.)

I also began to suffer with sinus issues and allergies— which had never surfaced in the past. A few sinus infections snuck in along the way. I can recall several 'episodes' where I had such a headache and such facial pain, plus my nose just running like a tap. No matter what I did with myself, relief was scarce. I remember lying down on the floor in tears, in the middle of the night on a couple of occasions.

These issues were bearable and whilst significantly annoying, never bad enough to seek medical intervention.

And so life took me to 2001, when I was aged 33 years.

## WELCOME TO THE WORLD CHENOA

On the 16th April 2001 at approx. 8:20pm, our beautiful daughter Chenoa was born—albeit 5 weeks early! Chenoa was delivered via caesarean section, due to breech position. Chenoa's conception and my pregnancy was smooth sailing and a wonderful experience. However I became concerned a few weeks before she was born, as I thought she had stopped moving. Several tests were performed and I was sent home and advised all was well, however she had not yet 'turned' into the correct position. My intuition proved correct. Upon admission to hospital on the day of her birth we were then informed that she had wedged herself quite firmly up under my ribs and would not have been able to move. Turning her in utero was not going to be a possibility, due to her position.

It was most important that she arrived safely with minimal trauma, so none of this bothered us—we just had full faith that we were in good hands and all would be well. And it was! Minimal trauma and excellent APGAR birth scores and here was our beautiful baby girl! Although slightly jaundice, and quite small—Chenoa spent her first 36 hours in humidicrib. This was a little sad for me as a new mother, as I could only reach one hand in through to touch her—for this time.

Initial feeding was an issue—for both her and for me. Unfortunately, although medication was given my breast milk did not arrive sufficiently. Coupled with the fact that she was so tired and premmie—we endured some feeding difficulties early on.

I did persevere and express whatever breast milk I could and again that was Ok and I wasn't too concerned about that—what could I do about it really? However, what did become stressful was the incredibly difficult regime of feeding that followed. Chenoa had to be taught to 'suck' and this was done via finger sucking, and then syringe tube. Once we were home, it was a challenging procedure to perform—especially when one was on their own, with no help. To tape the small tube to ones pinkie finger and try to get her to suck on both, then fill the syringe/tube with milk. Due to her prematurity and size—this needed to be done every 3 hours initially. Again, we coped & didn't give it too much thought—many people go through such challenges with premature and sick babies.

However, our little Chenoa faced many of her own challenges and setbacks, illnesses and issues in her early years—of which I will not go into in great detail, but suffice to say a whole other book could be written.

Now, this took its toll on me. But, at the time I was hearing all the comments that well-meaning people make, and that all this was 'normal' etc etc—but found I wasn't coping very well. It is only now when I look back and realise that if these challenges with baby Chenoa had existed in isolation then that would have possibly been OK.

However, in the back lines there were other things going on in my body and my own physical health was slowly declining and that made it hard for me to cope. These added stressors had more of an impact than thought at the time.

When Chenoa was 10 months old, we spent some time in 'Torrens House' (CAFHS—Child & Adolescent Family Health Service residential support service), for support and to address some of her sleep issues. Since her birth, sleep had been erratic—due to other problems she was encountering (but not diagnosed until she was aged over 2 years). From approx. 6 months of age, she began waking more often and became increasingly unsettled. For quite a few months, she was only sleeping for approx. 40 mins straight—both day and night (again there were reasons for this but unknown to us at that time). Thus, my sleeping patterns began to suffer.

Up until Chenoa was born I was used to sleeping very soundly—up to 8 hours each night and woke up feeling refreshed and ready to greet the day. However, when her sleeping became very disruptive, then I became very sleep deprived. Again, in isolation maybe this could be manageable for short period of time, but with other FMS issues slowly creeping in, my body was feeling the challenge! So, it was not uncommon for me to take longer and longer to get to sleep—just fade into sleep—to be woken again . . . then, for a while my body seemed to say 'it's not even worth going to sleep'. Anxiety followed this as I was on edge, waiting for the crying to wake me up!

Consequently, my deep and sound sleeping style went way out the window! My sleep became very short lived and very light. I could hear a pin drop and never fell into the totally deep and restorative sleep that is essential—especially with a young baby/child. Those of you familiar with FMS would be aware that changes to sleep patterns/trouble sleeping are very closely co related to onset of full blown FMS.

After much work and intervention, Chenoa's sleep patterns and habits did improve to a satisfactory level, but unfortunately mine did not.

From approx. late 2002 (Chenoa was aged 18 months) I faced more frequent sinus and allergy issues, more frequent (and acute) sinus infections, more frequent upper respiratory tract infections (including repeated episodes of bronchitis). I almost lived constantly with the most annoying aggravating and irritating cough (to both myself and those around me), and many medicines and strategies were used—to no avail!

My weight rapidly increased (to 90 kilograms), I began to experience an annoyingly itchy scalp and scalp sores, felt constantly tired, encountered repeatedly swollen glands in my neck. I endured more mouth ulcers than usual.

To top all this off, as if I didn't feel bad enough about myself—my hair began to rapidly thin out. The quick fix solution to help me 'cope', was the offer of anti-depressants! However, I knew that whilst I was depressed, this low frame of mind was coming from a different place. I was only 'not coping' because no one was able to tell me why my body was struggling.

My GP referred me to a dermatologist, who ran a heap of tests and undertook a scalp biopsy. No clear answers were given. I also consulted a 'trichologist', who advised me of *scalp psoriasis* and put me onto some shampoos and conditioners that would help manage (minimise) the scratching. But, no one found anything of significance in regards to my hair thinning out. I often left my GP scratching his head and he repeated several times blood tests to check my thyroid function and iron levels. I know that he felt quite certain that this was the 'problem', that caused my hair loss and my weight gain.

It is now known that whilst my T4 (thyroid hormone) level was 'borderline/low' and my TSH ('thyroid Stimulating Hormone') level was over '3' (late 2002)—this was within 'acceptable range'. However, had I been able to play this scenario again, I would have persuaded him to begin me on trial basis—for thyroid replacement therapy or suitable intervention. The other hormone tests performed were also 'within normal range'. I have also since read that if TSH level is greater than '2', then thyroid intervention/treatment is recommended—to avoid this getting to extreme state—which is of course what in fact unfolded for me at later date (2007).

I began addressing my weight and joined Weight Watchers at the beginning of 2004, after my weight reached 90 kilograms. My goal weight of 68 kilograms (highest end of healthy BMI range) was successfully achieved by the end of 2004! This program enabled me to focus on my weight loss and was practical and easy to follow. It took a lot of hard work, dedication and exercise—as there was still other factor why weight management was an issue (for me). I was very proud to achieve my goal weight; however, it was like trying to hold back the tide. I did not remain at my goal weight easily, as still one of the problematic metabolic issues was not addressed until 2008.

So, not only was a metabolic problem in existence that meant my weight wouldn't remain stable, there would have been more physical pressure from significant weight gain (up to 18 kilograms over 2 year timeframe)—followed by significant weight loss (20+ kgs within 11 months).

So, this is a snapshot of my 'pre diagnosis' symptoms and struggles. I knew that my body was not functioning as it should, but what can you do when you are to some degree 'at the mercy' of the medical profession. I should have pushed harder, and I know that now—and that has influenced my experiences in the period of 2007 to 2011. But, at that time, I was juggling motherhood, paid work (only approx.15 hours per week total) and home life. I began to believe that the 'problem' was me and that I wasn't coping as I was 'depressed'. I did give in for a short period of time—and went on anti-depressants (for approx. 9

months). Whilst they did settle some of the anxiety, I feel sure they also contributed to the weight gain. The 'niggling' things within my body continued and I held resolve and trust in myself that there was more to this picture than depression.

But, I also accepted that we had had a rough time with Chenoa's early years, and I think the anti-depressants together with the Professional counselling I received, did help me come to terms with some of these difficulties. However, I only went on the anti-depressants as a short term solution (support) and to satisfy those around me, and then went off them when I thought things were once again more manageable. I felt quite confident that my depression was 'reactive depression'.

When Chenoa was 3 years old and I felt things had stabilised a little with her health (in 2004), I made a major decision to leave my place of employment and have some mother—daughter bonding time with Chenoa at home, before she started kindergarten and (later) school. This was one of the best decisions I have ever made, and this time together was most enjoyable and will be treasured by me forever! Brenton fully supported this decision and so we went down to one income, but it was so worth it! Needless to say, all the same physical issues remained for me (in the background)—but I just got on with it, as I just wanted to enjoy our daughter and the precious time together.

When Chenoa started kindergarten, I recommenced my volunteer work (a few hours per week); and complemented this with part time/casual work to help support our household income. My paid work was mainly out of hours and thus Brenton was able to take care of Chenoa in my absence. This did restrict and reduce our 'family' time together, but it did work to our advantage for a while. My voluntary role led me back into permanent part time employment, back in community services again—and into a job that I loved (within Carer Support) and undertook with passion! This was able to be managed within kindergarten hours, and then school hours once Chenoa started school.

## Chapter Three

# The 'Crash' That Led To Diagnosis

In May 2007 I changed employment. I started in a new position at different workplace, same role but with a slight increase in hours (went up from 13 hours/week up to 20 hours/week total). This employment change was a new challenge for me. I threw myself into it and was thrilled with the different opportunities that were presented with the change.

I was given a lot of autonomy and my new colleagues had great belief in me (my abilities) and confidence in what I may be able to achieve, based on my previous Professional experience!

As with every year—the weeks between August and October were always most challenging for my immune system. With increased pollen activity, came increased allergies and it seemed my immune system had trouble dealing with this, resulting in sinus infections or other viruses and upper respiratory tract infections, which seemed to follow the winter. However, in 2007 I encountered a very significant episode of what began as *acute* **respiratory illness**—we thought it was just flu like illness. However, the physical effects of this episode were far reaching.

One night after work I put myself to bed early—feeling very poorly. I had the worst headache ever, together with high temperatures, chills, and an extremely achy body. I couldn't even sit up, due to headache and dizziness. Paracetamol had no affect and after a few hours still feeling unwell, I decided I needed something stronger. I never take strong medications unless in diabolic situation, as they have a tendency to make me feel very sick and sometimes even vomit. If I take a strong medication, I need to then go to sleep.

(I had been prescribed a stronger pain killer in the months before—in an effort to try to stop the unrelenting and never ending cough. I could only take it at bedtime, but it did help with the coughing.)

What I haven't mentioned to many people, is that on that night when I was trying to get sleep and obtain some relief I was actually afraid. I was afraid to go to sleep; afraid I would need to get up to be sick, afraid that I wouldn't wake up.

I did wake up—and approx. 6/7 hours had passed since taking the strong pain relief. Although still feeling a little poorly, I got out of bed and headed into the shower, having decided that I would assess how I coped in the shower—as to if I would be capable of going to work. I didn't feel like I still had high temperature, although I still felt bad—I didn't feel as unwell as I had the night before. I thought maybe I was suffering after affects from the stronger medication. Into the shower I go. The most overwhelming dizziness ensued and my body just went completely limp and the weirdest feeling went through my body—like a tornado.

I have fainted before but this was quite a different experience. I can remember feeling like I was paralysed but couldn't do anything with my body. I remember calling out to Brenton and feeling scared but blacked out. Ended up I collapsed onto the floor (like dead weight), but on the way down, managed to fall out of the shower and onto the hard ensuite door—putting a big hole into it. I don't remember anything until I realised I was flat out on the ground, completely wet, shower still running and just couldn't get up.

Eventually Brenton and Chenoa managed to get me up and back into bed. Brenton took care of things that morning and called my work to tell them I wouldn't be in. I insisted I was OK, and consequently he took our daughter with him to work, and left the phone with me—just in case. I still felt dizzy, and sick—couldn't move my head. I also couldn't 'feel' my body and was very scared that I couldn't move. About 30 minutes after they had left the house—I still didn't feel any better and decided to call an ambulance. I became concerned that I had received a blow to my head and maybe should get things checked out.

Brenton was none the wiser at this point, and the ambulance arrived within approx. 15 mins (as it was non urgent), checked me out, questioned me, struggled to get me onto their stretcher and took me off to hospital. They had agreed that it was all a little unusual and seemed to be concerned that I had experienced some kind of seizure.

In the hospital emergency department I still couldn't move—as I thought I'd throw up. They put monitors on me, ran some tests, put a drip in and all I can remember is that they were fussing and I just wanted to sleep and escape from how I was feeling! A few hours later, they had found nothing concrete but were a little confused by what had happened. They kept me in for observation for the next 12 hours, due to extremely low blood pressure and stated they wouldn't let me go home until this rectified. They also ran more blood tests and advised me to follow up the results with my GP within the next 24 hours—as well as follow up.

Mysteriously it is still unknown why these events unravelled but the chances are it was in fact some type of seizure activity. Apart from the continuing extremely low blood pressure, my white cell count was also extremely low, and cortisol levels were extremely high—due to stress my body was under. The pain in my body really started from that morning. I began to encounter ongoing episodes of pins and needles all through my body. I was also extremely shaky for days afterwards.

This low blood pressure continued for weeks and I felt flat, however my GP (at that time) just put it all down to a virus, and again didn't really HEAR my concerns nor connect the dots. I spoke with a good friend at that time and she acknowledged my anxiety and fear and she suggested a **second opinion from another doctor**. She recommended her GP of whom she spoke highly, and stated how thorough he was and explained to me how he looked into things beyond the 'norm'.

So, I called him and had my first appointment approx. 4 weeks after the 'mystery shower incident'. I explained to him how exhausted my body had been since then—like it had run 10 marathons and was trying to recover. His first 'plan of attack' based on the 'presenting history', was to order more blood tests. He included all hormones and thyroid function tests. Tests were done and follow up with him resulted in a referral to an endocrinologist specialist, and a further few months went by whilst I awaited this appointment.

In January (2008) I started to document my pain and symptoms, as I thought it may help with the specialist consultation. The pain within my body was described as 'migratory pain'. My neck and head were included in the pain that was experienced. I described the pain in the following ways (over the next 3-4 months)—

'dull deep ache'—so intense in elbow that it took strength away in arm

Very sore-like dead weights

'sore legs, buttocks, ache in toes, knee'

Weakness in Left hand side arm

Knee throbbing

Hip aching

Sore legs, achy front and back

Knees, toes, wrist, ankle throbbing pain

Deep burning pain, stabbing pain, knife turning pain.

As well as this hard to explain pain, I also began to experience 'overwhelming exhaustion'.

At all times, there was pain somewhere in my body, joints, shoulders, head, neck.

My sleep became erratic due to discomfort. Sometimes the pain would be extremely intense and other times would be throbbing pain. A physio diagnosed **bursitis** in my upper thighs.

NSAID's (Non-steroidal Anti Inflammatory Drugs) were taken some nights, as well as paracetamol to try and manage the pain spasms. Headaches were increasing, as was the tiredness and fatigue.

Energy levels and stamina was decreasing and periods of EXTREME fatigue were increasing by the day. The higher the physical demand was on my body = the more significant was the pain. My body also became sore to the slightest touch. I couldn't lift my daughter due to weakness.

The (small, pea sized) gland in my neck was also up and down—would remain swollen/raised for weeks on end, then 'normal'. I almost always had a sore throat and often had mouth ulcers. My sleep continued to deteriorate. I began to become breathless upon minimal exertion. Hanging out washing, making beds were hard to bear and near impossible. Needless to say the shopping, vacuuming and activities requiring higher exertion level were very difficult and left me exhausted and in pain.

I felt like just sitting in the chair all day, every day. I struggled to move and engage in any aspects of daily living, and didn't want to. Some days, when not working I would do just that—sit, in a chair, in my own company—for hours. BUT, it didn't make me feel any better! Any sleep I did manage to get—was not refreshing. I woke still feeling exhausted—thus never ready to face the next day!

I became increasingly anxious, and nervy, shaky, lost appetite, and started to get very vague—like I couldn't think. I became confused very easily and multi-tasking went out the window! I had to really concentrate to concentrate.

I was now **very** sensitive to lights and sounds at shops etc and felt 'out of contact' (dreaming) when in those environments. I could only manage very short periods, if at all. My appetite decreased, my blood pressure was low. My hair thinning continued and caused much distress. My vision changed almost on daily basis—I had optometrist appointments—check of visual factors, visual field etc. I lost confidence driving and driving at night (as well as going out at night) just became too stressful.

I was experiencing severe sinus through the night and would wake up feeling as if I was unable to breathe—due to being blocked up! This was known as 'travelling nocturnal sinus congestion', and I could feel it move from one side to the other side, as I switched my sleeping sides! It could be described as 'a swishing of water'.

Now, I acknowledge that many people experience difficult symptoms and periods of time—with all the above symptoms. However, for me (and others with Fibromyalgia), these symptoms often occurred all at the same time—and didn't really stop for any more than a few minutes at a time. For relatively short periods of time, most things are tolerable—but when you experience sleep issues AS WELL AS the other symptoms/ issues—on an ongoing basis for not just weeks but months on end—it does start to become aggravating indeed!

Due to the referral(s) to the specialist(s), I was documenting my symptoms—to assist with the initial consultations—with the endocrinologist and the rheumatologist. My symptoms and pain became quite significant as did my anxiety levels whilst I was awaiting these appointments—as I struggled to make sense of what was happening. My intolerance to hot and cold accelerated. My body temperatures were all over the place—with no appearing pattern or logic.

I was becoming easily confused and lost concentration ability. My memory ability changed. Even now, I try to be systematic with where I put things but still often have no recollection and take extensive time to recall. People have constantly brushed it off as being forgetful and that they also experience this. However, my mind and memory used to be sharp as a tack. I could remember phone numbers, registration plates, and birthdays. Although I am a little better than when first struggling with FMS, this is still challenging for me. And given what I was like in this area, for many years—I now experience a frustrating and stark contrast. Paying bills, remembering things, concentrating, and understanding some processes are now actions that require intense concentration. Sometimes I have trouble with words, and know what I mean but either use the wrong word, or cannot think of the word at all. Even driving sometimes requires strict concentration and a lot more 'energy'.

I remember one day I went into the Adelaide CBD as I was meeting a couple of friends for lunch. I had to work out where to park and how to get there. At that time, I used to have to write down the floor level and any reminder prompts to find the car again afterwards. Then, I had to somehow walk from the car to the designated lunch venue. All went well until the fatigue set in after the lunch. I amazingly returned to the car (remembered where it was) and absently started the car and knew I was going home. But, next thing I realised I was actually driving 'up' the ramp to higher levels, although I knew I had to go down in my logical mind.

My initial consult with endocrinologist was in December 2007 and was 'interesting', but more about this 'chapter' in my journey a little later. I wasn't able to keep records from blood results, as this specialist wasn't keen to share and I wasn't of clear thinking mind at that time. I was extremely easily confused and the simplest tasks were challenging—for example, coping with paying the specialist bills and working out what to do with Medicare etc.

During my first visit I was diagnosed with 'premature ovarian failure' and ('synthetic HRT') medication began. Whilst this specialist was 'interested' in my reflex response and pain—was totally focussed on blood levels of hormones and his intention was simply to rectify these levels. However, from my recollection, my hypothyroidism was not treated (medicated) until approx. 3 months later (and within weeks on the medication a gallbladder attack ensued around middle of April—resulting in gall bladder removal). Thus, whilst some answers were provided, I remained hopeful that my initial consultation with the rheumatologist may give me more answers and information. According to my documentation, the thyroid medication did initially provide some slight improvement to fatigue and exhaustion. I continued to struggle through and did the best I could, until my gall bladder was removed on 22nd May (2008). Finally my consultation with the next specialist Mid June 2008!

I struggled to cope with both the physical and emotional stress at work throughout this period of 'waiting time' of more than 6 months. I became breathless very easily. I also increasingly struggled with social events and interacting took its toll, I found solace in 'down time' and enjoyed alone time, as it didn't demand energy of me that I didn't have. Stress had a huge impact and I would become very overwhelmed when confronted with too many demands or things to think about. My coping ability to stress became extremely low and depleted.

On the 20th June 2008 the rheumatologist specialist undertook a thorough examination. He asked questions in follow up to the questionnaires I had completed prior, and spent some time listening to my explanation and description of what had unfolded in the 9 months prior to this appointment. His diagnosis was 'Fibromyalgia'. He provided some information on the condition, suggested some management techniques, and suggested my consideration of some long term pain management medications. He suggested that my decisions (about medication options) be followed up with my GP.

A whole new era had just begun in my journey for answers and explanations. In some ways, the diagnoses I had been given by both specialists were reassuring and provided a huge amount of temporary relief. They validated the pain and symptoms I had been experiencing. Both of these specialists had made suggestions and started some medication regimes. So, I followed their suggestions and began the waiting game, until my next visit with endocrinologist in August 2008.

At this next visit, results of blood tests were not given nor discussed with me—but changes were made by increasing dosages of the medications. I attempted to inform this specialist that I didn't yet feel any improvements and was still struggling with the same issues and symptoms and was not yet feeling any 'better'. I was offered increased doses, and in addition to this—offered anti-depressants. This was because according to this specialist the blood results 'had improved' and thus my health status had 'improved', even though I was suggesting otherwise. This meant, to him—that the next step was anti-depressants!

I was absolutely devastated, distressed, frustrated and so disappointed! I left that visit in tears, and immediately telephoned my GP (didn't even leave the car park), to advise him that I had no intention of returning to this specialist and made a follow up appointment with the GP. Nearly 12 months had transpired at that point, since my original 'system crash'! Apart from my gall bladder incident I had not been having regular appointments with this GP.

This changed at that point! I had spent 12 months waiting on doctors' appointments, going from one appointment to the next, whilst also trying to work, function as best I could, and run the household—needless to say, the exhaustion didn't help but somehow I managed to drag myself through this 'limbo' time. And, after all this, I didn't feel any better than 12 months before—even though I had been following the treatment protocols and medications and that was very disheartening.

My GP was absolutely wonderful and has been ever since! I informed him what had gone on, what I had discovered and what I had been told by the specialist(s). He saw my distress and I asked him straight out if he could treat me from that point—and no one else! I was tired of consulting different doctors for different things and felt like I wasn't actually making any progress—like each of them were only treating 'their little part' of the complex 'whole system'. I wanted to be treated in holistic sense, and listened to and offered respect and compassion. I didn't have the energy nor wish to spend every second of time (that I wasn't at work) attending appointments that really were not very productive! But, I guess it was also a process of elimination and logically I knew and understood that—but it didn't make this time any easier!

My wonderful GP has from that point (to this day) tried to address my state of health in a more holistic way. From the start he has worked 'with me' and not 'for me'. We have addressed my health and state of wellbeing together. I have cried with him, he has encouraged me. We have laughed together and he has boosted my coping abilities.

He has offered reassurance along the way. He has validated my experiences, whilst also looking beyond blood results and acknowledged me 'the patient' and treated ME and not just the results.

He has always sent me away from my visits feeling like I AM able to keep going. He has been honest and told me that it's a very slow process. But, he has also told me how well I have managed to get to this point. He has praised me for how I have continued moving forward in such trying circumstances. He has helped me more than he would know.

At that visit his action is what made all the difference to me. He asked me 'what I wanted to do next' and 'how did I want to proceed from here'. He included me in the outcome and put me into the centre of the situation—he put the balance of power back where it needed to be! That is, an equal relationship between a health Professional and a client (patient). My confidence was renewed after being so crushed! So, forwards we went—in collaboration.

Initially it was a complete turnaround with medications and treatment—as he had listened to my concerns. I advised him that although I had been put on medications and 'should' have improved and 'should' be feeling better—the bottom line was that I WAS NOT feeling any better than I was 12 months prior! We began a new regime, beginning with completely new blood work—which revealed what I had intuitively known. The hormone levels had deteriorated significantly, except for TSH and T4 (Thyroid) levels, which had improved BUT dosages still required change—for further improvement.

Within less than 4 months (on this new regime) I experienced some improvements with blood (hormone) levels, and even the thyroid levels had seemed to stabilise. My moods had stabilised (partly due to switching to Bio identical HRT), the headaches had decreased, as had the confusion.

I was coping a little better with stress and was coping overall much better (than when at my worst). However, exhaustion and pain was still significant. My sleep was assisted by the new medication(s). I began to feel 'like there was light at the end of the tunnel'.

Since then and along the way, the next 2 years involved changes to medications and changes to dosages—attempting to get appropriate levels. Again my weight became problematic but I was addressing it accordingly. We cautiously tried new things, and he addressed any concerns I had in a courteous and respectful manner. Early 2010 my blood tests and GP visits were stretched out to 3 monthly (from 2 monthly), as results and my management had stabilised to satisfactory level. Early in 2011, the blood tests and GP visits went to six monthly! What an exciting achievement that was!

Earlier in my struggles it had been suggested several times by concerned friends and colleagues, the possibility of seeking input from a Naturopath. Unfortunately I didn't think this was possible at that time—as things were too 'unstable'. However, much to my surprise (and delight) my GP suggested I may benefit from this type of Practitioner, in May 2010—

once some of my issues had 'stabilised'. Not only did he make the suggestion—he also offered a referral to one that he was working with. I again felt very lucky to have such an open minded GP who valued the benefits of working in collaboration—not just with the patient but also with other Practitioners.

So, since May 2010 I have been consulting both of these Health Professionals and they work just wonderfully together and appear to have a sound Professional Relationship based on mutual respect. Together they are working to achieve the best possible outcome(s) for their patients with their 'Integrated Approach'.

The Naturopath has offered assistance that has greatly assisted my health whilst complementing the GP and his intervention(s). I have no doubt that this combination has greatly enabled me to get to where I have and achieve such stable management of my physical condition. Together, we are learning and aiming for good outcomes that benefit my health.

I have also been pursuing with keen interest the benefits of nutritional medicine. And so, in many regards the journey for improved physical health (restoring) still continues.

It has been a very long, frustrating and tiresome road to travel. But, I am grateful that I have had the fortunate experience of having a few wonderful people assisting me. It has made a remarkable difference to where I am, and what we have been able to achieve. Sometimes the people that we expect will be around to support and assist us are nowhere to be seen, or for various reasons, are unable to be of assistance in our time of need. Then out of the sidelines appear other people that are able to guide us along. These people appear when we least expect it but we need to keep hope that the right help will be there for us.

More information will be disclosed and shared, about these valuable people a little later (in part Two) when I describe 'My team of health Professionals'.

## Chapter Four

# Important Decisions In 2011

In April 2011, I resigned from my position after 4 and half years, working 20 hours/week. Various stressors prompted this resignation.

Contributing stress in the workplace took its toll, on top of the ongoing management of FMS. In (late) 2010, my health and wellbeing had improved and blood test results had stabilised to satisfactory levels. The results (Thyroid function and hormones) were where I had aimed to be for quite a while. In March 2011, my GP advised me that I didn't need another appointment for 6 months—or blood tests for 6 months! Finally, stable and managed—although still work to be done with the Naturopath.

Leading up to April 2011 stress in the workplace had slowly crept up over a 6 month period, until I didn't feel that I was able to manage the conflicting demands—as well as my health issues and our family life. Again, FMS had contributed to a situation that was possibly able to be managed (to most people) however, increased physical and emotional stress has significant impacts on a person with FMS. My decision to resign was not easy (as I had a great passion for my work, including a strong commitment to the Carers), but I knew I had to do what was right for me. The decision made was based on supporting and maintaining my health whilst managing my stress levels. I had to make a choice—to make progress. We discussed this at length as a family and then followed through with the decision.

It is unlikely that I will be able to work full time within the next few years. It may be a possibility that in the future I will be able to work part time again. However, this will be dependent on many factors and will greatly depend on how my FMS management is going. I will need to be mindful of suitable options that remain flexible and allow me to utilise time when I feel more positive and energetic (currently between 10am and 2pm) and allow time to recharge when needed. As I also need to balance our home life and the needs of our family (and the extra energy needed for this, due to FMS)—it's likely I will only cope with minimal hours to best manage in long term.

There have been other stress factors that come from managing on one income. But these do not have such a dramatic impact on my condition (and wellbeing), as the physical stress and impacts from the many demands that come with working a 20 hour working week, **plus** household and family responsibilities, **on top of** managing a chronic condition. We have to make choices and decisions that relate to our lifestyle, spending and personal situation. However, the physical stress of balancing finances, relationships, school life, domestic chores, shopping, banking, cleaning (and everything else) is significant and sufficient—without adding to the mix the added pressure that work routines can bring (early mornings, packing lunches, school pick-ups, coping with sickness and so on). Another person facing similar issues may make quite different choices and these will be right for them. We should refrain from judging another for their choices, as we are all doing the best we can.

Earlier in 2011, I again felt completely and extremely exhausted by the time I reached my workplace at 9am! Then as other situations arose in the workplace, I would become quite overwhelmed (exhausted) and struggle to get through the day—every day.

By the time we got home from school at 3:30 in the afternoon, I was too exhausted to deal with anything else—but pushed on, from necessity—to get tea, help with homework etc. Albeit, mostly not very well.

I felt I owed more to our daughter, as well as our home life. She deserved more support with her schooling and should enjoy her time away from school—with some activities and opportunities. She should not miss out on too much of life—due to this condition. So, now I am more able to structure my weekdays to better support her—assist with homework, care for her when she's sick and provide guidance through difficulties as they arise in her life—without finding it overwhelming. As we are also self-employed with a small business, the household was under too much stress and the effort needed to get through each week was taking its toll. Every ounce of energy was gone on the absolute necessary chores and responsibilities, and nothing was left over for anything else!

I felt very compelled upon first leaving my employment (April 2011) to catch up on things at home. Since I became unwell in 2007, it became harder for us to sustain the status quo on the home front. I relied more heavily on Brenton and we followed a pattern of low key weekends, to help us to cope. We did what we needed to do and not much more. We didn't get to take family holidays and our only breaks from home and 'life' were at (our caravan) Victor Harbor.

Resigning from work enabled me to take my time, and get some chores done that had not had much attention for 4 years. It also enabled me to focus on improving our quality of life—within our financial capacity. To plan and book some family holidays. To feel like I can manage to find energy to go on some family holidays is a huge bonus. To re connect with some people socially. To re connect with extended family, after many years of 'disconnection', as well as wonderful friends from school days. To make some amazing new connections and friendships!

To escape feeling exhausted and then feeling guilty—for not being able to fulfil the responsibilities that are important to me. To review some financial matters, insurances etc. To take some time to focus on my own spirituality. To feel like I am no longer living permanently in *fight-flight* mode, and running on adrenaline every single minute of every single day of every week. To put some energy into nutrition and eating better. To put some energy into exercise. To focus on my holistic wellbeing. To write—and therefore, do some healing.

September 2011 again brought into our home our share of sickness. Swine Flu/H1N1 hit us pretty hard and we still had things to deal with—for me the secondary issues of acute significant sinus infection and bronchitis set me back in many ways.

Life happens, and we all have our share of ups and downs but I didn't get so overwhelmed when these things cropped up—as there was less weight on my shoulders. I feel calmer and more grounded than I have for a long time—not quite so overwhelmed!

I still battle with many of the same things but exercise helps, as does my Professional Team of my GP and Naturopath, and family. I would not hesitate to seek out a psychologist (again) if the need was to arise. Medications assist me, and are complemented by natural (gentle) remedies and supplements where possible—from my wonderful Naturopath! Blood test results are overall quite stable—but sometimes we still struggle with some of these.

My body (and liver) seem to be coping with the medications and we now need to monitor the possibility of side effects and/or increased risk factors—as result of utilising some of the medications. However, all I can do is weigh up the pros and cons and make an informed decision at the time I need to.

Currently, my GP and I are discussing the possibility of again undertaking a 'cycle' of growth hormone, via daily injection. This may increase my IGF-1 levels and increase my energy levels. But, due to the cost and that we are now on one income, I will postpone this until later in 2012. The 'fine tuning' that we will still tackle may increase my energy and blood levels and improve my sense of wellness but the key is maintaining a good level of well-being. This requires a different set of tools and equipment, as well as lifestyle changes.

I still have pain and episodes of extreme fatigue, every day. But have learnt to live with it and do what I can to keep within my pain and energy threshold. To accept that I need to change plans, and do what I need to do—when I need to do it. To know that I need to listen to my body and not feel guilty. To accept that I am the one that lives with this stuff day in and day out and I KNOW what I need to do, to get through—as well as to keep a smile on my face, to keep some happiness, to maintain my wellbeing. I need to dedicate energy to myself and then I can remain positive and achieve better results with those around me the most.

We are all interconnected—like a jigsaw. But the most important pieces that are needed in the beginning before we can extend the jigsaw—are the pieces that fit closest. That's the ones who are nearest and dearest to us—usually our family and loved ones. These need to be our initial focus and responsibility. But, before that there is the initial starting point—this is ourselves. Before we can extend outwards, add to or build the puzzle we must be sure of our start point. OUR SELF is the very first piece and must be the starting point! We need to love ourselves enough to provide our own nurturing and then we may begin to HEAL, from the inside. Our first responsibility is to our own health and then we may begin to extend in a more productive way—outwards, to others closest to us.

The foundation of any family needs a good, firm and solid base—from which to grow—and also to face change and overcome challenges. This foundation is also influenced by the lifestyle of the family. Many other important factors also determine the 'family'.

The family unit is influenced by the members, who each bring their own strengths and individuality. Some family units are 'exciting, social, hectic'. We should refrain from envy, as we can never be certain what 's going on within that family and what influences and factors are coming into play for that family. (Ours may be described as 'stable, calm, low key'.)

Our family brings 3 very different personalities and sets of values. But we have many similarities and obviously have shared values. Brenton, Chenoa and myself are very much individuals, but we strengthen each other and have together, through our shared experiences built a firm foundation for our family. As result of FMS, Chenoa will have very different experiences (and opportunities) to many of her peers.

They will not be better or worse—they will just be HERS. Her character will be built from her view of the world, her experiences, her family and her support networks. If nothing else, I will have shared with her a very strong view that it is our inner strength that builds our strength of character.

Each and every one of us should stand proud of their character that has been made rich by FMS. We acquire a depth and an understanding of sympathy, empathy and compassion. These are all positive character aspects. FMS provides opportunities for richness and depth, however it is our character that determines the tools we will need and how much opportunity we allow ourselves!

I now encourage you to read on to PART TWO of this book. This will offer some suggestions, words of encouragement and I will share some of the strategies I have tried, some useful resources that have assisted me. Remember to keep in mind that I do not recommend anything in particular but simply share *my experiences*. I offer this with the intention that this may assist you, offer hope and encouragement or enlighten you in some way.

FMS is very complex and we are all unique people, but the best thing you can do for yourself is remain open minded and NEVER ever give up hope that the light will appear at the end of the tunnel. You will find your own light—you will go down that tunnel and light that lantern yourself! However, you will need to search for your own answers within yourself— unfortunately there is no 'quick fix' or easy solution. Your biggest asset and source of strength is actually within yourself. I hope that you will understand the importance and meaning of this a little better—by the end of PART TWO . . .

# PART TWO

*'What Lies behind us and what lies in front of us are small matters, compared to what lies within us'. (Ralph Waldo Emerson)*

It is said by many Professionals that Fibromyalgia Syndrome is a **'Syndrome'** of symptoms and challenges within the body which result as manifestations of a poorly functioning hypothalamus. (A 'multi system' disorder!). In my opinion, it is critical that we adopt a multi system approach, and encompass our healing on many levels and adopt a wide, integrative understanding—as well as a complementary approach, that addresses factors from a Pharmalogical and also Non Pharmalogical perspective. Do your own research and ask many questions—of others with this condition, and also the 'experts' in their areas of expertise. Also choose very carefully where you spend your money!

## CHAPTER ONE

# MY TEAM OF HEALTH PROFESSIONALS

## 1/ MY GP

For the years before 2007, I had a GP I had been happy with. Still to this day, in the case of acute illness I would not hesitate to take myself or other family members to be treated by him. However, around the time of the 'big episode' in 2007 it became clear that what was going on physically for me required knowledge in specific areas, that prompted me to seek a second opinion. This second opinion needed to be from a doctor who was well informed, and in many ways—whose knowledge equated to that of a consulting 'physician'. I have no doubt that had I not sought a second opinion at that time, I would have continued to remain in 'poor health'.

From the initial consultation with my current GP, I felt confident that his knowledge and expertise along with his commitment to patients' good health meant that I was now in good care. He seemed to have a particular interest in 'the challenge' at hand. Whilst it has been a 'game' of blood results, levels, increasing/decreasing doses it has also been about 'how I am feeling', and where possible—connecting the two together. If this wasn't possible, then we continued looking for other explanations.

I was able to express my concerns and how my physical health was impacting on my quality of life. According to my journal THE THINGS THAT WORRIED ME (as at March 2008) were—

Reduced Quality of life (reduced capacity, stamina)
Not feeling like doing things—too exhausted
Fatigue
Getting puffed out
Feeling vague
Not sleeping
Feeling overwhelmed
Red 'surface' rash-feeling anxious when under stress
The migratory pain—constantly present!

All of these factors were also combined with the uncertainty and lack of understanding about what was happening with my physical health and to my state of mind.

By September 2008 I had tried a range of different strategies to help me cope with this uncertainty and my levels of anxiety. We witnessed only slow stabilisation of blood results and often I would be reminded how we were dealing with some 'fine tuning' and there was no quick fix. That it was going to take time, and we could only make a certain number of changes at any one time. Tests were done on anything that was related to the metabolic systems and energy production systems.

From my reading and researching it was suggested many times that FMS is closely related to deficits (under functioning) in the hypothalamus-pituitary-adrenal gland (HPA) axis.

Although my GP knew what my official 'diagnosis' had been, we never attached our 'game plan' to any one condition (diagnosis). We tried to avoid the 'labelling' of the conditions, as it was plain to see that in my case the issues were to do with 'multi systems', and each had a trickle effect on another. Still to this day, I don't really know if my GP attached the term 'fibromyalgia' to my poor health. However, whether he is aware of it or not he has followed some text book intervention offered by one of the most helpful books on FMS that I have ever read.

Jacob Teitelbaum's wonderful book '**From Fatigued To Fantastic**'(2007) focuses on his main outcome—

to move from fatigue to wellness. He travelled this journey himself, and understands that comprehensive medicine is needed to address the syndrome of symptoms. Teitelbaum explains FMS in broader sense as manifestations of a poorly functioning hypothalamus, and that perhaps the underlying problems (poor health) lead to an energy crisis within the body.

He considers that a range of factors are in play—infections (immune dysfunctions), nutritional deficiencies, hormonal imbalances and these all have the ability to either trigger or perpetuate FMS. It is a possibility that as soon as sleep problems or disruptions arise, the FMS may become 'self-perpetuating'. The influence of the sleep issue can suppress the hypothalamus. This fabulous book makes use of his own SHINE protocol, and he suggests strategies and ways to work through—'S'leep, 'H'ormone imbalances, 'I'nfections, 'N'utrition, 'E'xercise.

Although I had never discussed this book or regime with my GP—over the course of time he has systematically addressed these issues with me. To start with the issue of SLEEP, we have to ascertain if it is sleep maintenance or the falling to sleep/ returning to sleep that is the main issue. In my case, it was taking me around 45 mins (average) to get to sleep, and would wake after approx. 3 hours—

then take around an hour to get back to sleep—for another 2 hours before it was time to rise for the day. Even when I slept for block of 2 or 3 hours, it was extremely light sleep and I would wake at slightest sound or disturbance. This was stark contrast to the solid 8 hours sleep per night I was used to. (The deep sleep states are necessary for tissue repair and for the release of Human Growth Hormone.)

We tried a couple of different sleep aids to encourage sleep restoration and these assisted with the management of the pain that prevented sleep (including bursitis on each thigh).

I tried sleeping tablets and eventually ENDEP together with sinus sprays to assist with night time sinus. I also did my own endless research (regarding sleep) and added a few of my own strategies (music, good sleep hygiene, yoga, mindfulness) and these will be discussed separately. The ENDEP combined with FESS spray initially gave me some good results. Once some sleep restoration occurred, other things also 'calmed' to a reasonable level. The ENDEP made me drowsy at bedtime but I didn't really get to sleep any quicker. Whilst I still woke through the night—it did assist me getting *back to sleep* quicker, thus less waking time through the night. I stayed on the ENDEP for approx. 5 months but then found that the other 'natural' alternatives assisted me enough to get through. Without the ENDEP my sleep pattern was then around 4 hours straight, usually 12 till 4 am.

I am sure stabilising other factors (hormonal) has also supported some improvements in the sleep regime. Now, I can usually have a stretch of light sleep of 6-7 hours, on approx. 4 nights of the week. I fall to sleep easier/quicker—mostly around 11:30pm and wake early in the morning on these nights. The remaining 2 or 3 nights of the week are a little more unsettled. There seems to be no set pattern or influencing factors but I currently cope OK with this, as long as I get short breaks/rests through the afternoon. No matter neither how much sleep I manage nor how solid this sleep is—I am still unrefreshed and unmotivated upon waking. I still feel tired and lethargic and my body feels 'heavy' in the morning. The best strategy for me is to remain in bed until approx. 8am, and then I feel a 'little' more able to face the day ahead. However, this is not possible very often due to daily commitments. Prior to my 30's I was refreshed and eager in the mornings. I was very motivated and ready to 'seize the day'.

HORMONAL factors opened a whole can of worms! After deciding I didn't intend to have the endocrinologist specialist on my TEAM, I commenced compounded Bio Identical HRT (which, for me compounds 4 hormones of varying doses into one 'troche'), to support some of the hormonal issues. As well as being advised that I was experiencing at that time 'secondary ovarian failure' (due to hypothalamus/pituitary issues)—it was also discovered that my thyroid was under functioning, and my adrenal glands were also struggling (thus also low levels of DHEA-S). My IGF1 (Insulin Growth Factor) levels were also low and are still low (equivalent to a 60 to 70 year old person!).

An MRI scan was also undertaken through this process, and it appears my pituitary is small in size—perhaps has shrunk, or was always small—but either way it seems to be under functioning, and not able to continue output of demand to meet my physical needs. For a while the term 'hypopituitarism' was used to assist my understanding, which was needed to accept what was needed next. What followed was a range of interventions that focussed on substituting/replacing the supply of the required hormones.

Upon researching I discovered that this began to make sense, as one of the main functions of the adrenal glands assist us with managing stress, which was an issue for me.

The low levels of IGF1 (Insulin Growth factor) may also have direct link to lack of energy and muscle weakness. Growth Hormone supports the immune system and helps the body fight off infection. Human Growth Hormone was delivered via daily injection for a few months, and this will be repeated again in near future—however there is a high cost for this replacement therapy. *ALSO prior to commencing Growth Hormone Replacement it is important to rule out the presence/possibility of Pituitary Tumours.*

I discovered (via my own researching) that Adrenal deficiency can possibly contribute to weight gain, tiredness, muscle and joint pain and insomnia. I also discovered it could possibly be linked with allergies, hair loss, circulation problems, fatigue, low stamina and low energy output. Of course it's also closely related to how well your body responds to stress—physical, emotional and psychological. The main connections are cortisol production and DHEA. Low cortisol production may mean a person drags themselves through the day—feeling exhausted. On the other hand, high cortisol levels may give people 'energy to burn' (adrenaline junkies).

If a person's adrenals are not producing sufficient hormones the end result may be that the person functions OK when things are stable—but if stress is added, they are unable to cope. The person with 'malfunctioning adrenal glands' may also be vulnerable to infections, suffer with headaches, and possibly with joint/muscle pain. Allergies or chemical sensitivities may arise OR may become worse. Many of these 'symptoms' overlap with other possible conditions (eg hypothyroidism), and sometimes both conditions occur together. However they are also both metabolic problems that result in a slowdown of body function and thus a decline in energy is the final outcome. With FMS the body is most often in 'stressed' state, as it struggles to manage.

Over the last few years and certainly to this day, I have developed and continue to have a very low threshold to cope with cold. I never used to experience this, and in Adelaide we do not experience extreme cold or long periods of cold climate. However, it is not uncommon for me to need up to 4 times the amount of 'added' warmth (especially at night). It is not unusual for me to wear socks to bed all year round. In the cooler months I also require flannelette PJ's, flannelette sheets plus a quilt and added 2 to 3 blankets plus either electric blanket or heat bag/source, where others may need the PJ's, the warmer sheets and a quilt.

Also, throughout this time along with exhaustion/fatigue, when I am at my worst and haven't slept well for more than a few nights, I also experience extreme nausea. When I am tired = nausea—which adds to the whole not feeling too great picture!

I often still experience limbs (legs, arms, feet) going 'to sleep'. Like when you cross your legs or arms and affect the circulation, and may find you can't feel these limbs when you go to stand or move. However, I do not need to aggravate my body by crossing my legs or sitting or standing in awkward positions. I may simply be watching TV at night, and after an hour I may go to get up and find that I have to wait for up to 10 mins before I get feeling to my feet, legs or arms. More noticeably legs and feet, as these are needed to walk/move. So, hopefully in time we will be able to identify and manage this issue a little better.

To add some positive light to these medical results and symptoms, I have regularly also had blood tests to monitor Liver Function (due to medication load), Iron, Ferritin, insulin and cholesterol and all have brought in good results!

Just in closing this section regarding my own GP. I have read widely many Practitioners saying that treating a person with FMS was quite different to many other patients that suffer from health problems such as cancer etc and other chronic problems (like migraines etc).

As people with FMS are often known as *Type A Over Achievers*, this also means they generally wish to be well informed, empowered and have a strong desire to understand what is happening to them and what may be available to them. They seek to be actively involved in the process and the pathways along the way.

In my case this has definitely been true! In my darkest and most acute times (of uncertainty and despair) I was rarely able to manage to read for more than 15-20 mins at a time, due to trouble concentrating and fatigue. This was out of character for me—after growing up with a passion for reading, a thirst for knowledge and a strong belief that 'knowledge is power'—which was reinforced whilst doing study and then Bachelor degree in 1998-2001.

But, I did what I could at the time. Every time we had test results, I would studiously record them in my book, whilst at my appointment. My GP would discuss what this result meant and/or what it may be indicative of, and how it connected with the bigger picture. I would then go home, research widely on the topic (or medication etc) and try to work out how we could address and connect with everything else that was going on.

Then, upon my next visit—which at that time was 6 to 8 weeks—I would present the GP with what I had found, we would discuss how we would then include this new information into our game plan/ strategy. My GP showed extreme patience with this behaviour. Needless to say I certainly learnt a lot about the human system.

I remember at one time, Brenton suggested to me that I must drive my GP crazy with how I was behaving. I hadn't even thought of this. It hadn't ever crossed my mind—because I had never picked up on any negativity. But, I remember I asked the GP at my next visit—probably just to reassure Brenton.

Basically, I questioned the GP outright, and said what Brenton had been thinking and asked him how he felt about my way of managing the logical side of my journey. My question went something like—

'Do I drive you crazy when I bring in all this information, and go off in search of information, and then question you about it all?'.

I will never forget he just looked at me and simply said

'Not at all. I think it's great that you want to learn more and understand what's happening. It's your way of making sense of it and coping. You are obviously a very intelligent, bright person and if this helps you in any way then please continue as you are doing'. He then looked at me and added 'And I need to remain open minded—as I don't know it all. Through this process you may in fact tell me something that I haven't considered and may be worth considering. We are learning as we go. Every person is different and you are entitled to keep your own power through this'.

This may not be his EXACT words, but I would bet you he wouldn't even remember that conversation. But, I nearly hugged him! His words had such an impact on me. But more than that, I thought (yet again)—'how lucky am I to have this amazing Doctor'!

In early 2010, my GP kindly offered a referral to a Naturopath, which was gladly accepted. These 2 Health Practitioners complement each other with their collaborative approach.

It was with this Naturopath, that the next elements 'I'nfections and 'N'utritional deficiencies were to be addressed. I am thankful for private Health Insurance, as without it I would not have been able to afford many of the 'extra' treatments and therapies that I sourced.

***This is your new reality. You choose the colour of your landscape.***

## 2/ NATUROPATH

The Naturopath complements my GP's work and one of the first things she did was review all my blood tests, and tried to link how I am feeling to how my body is dealing with waste, absorbing nutrients and breaking down foods. The gut has been a major part of this overhaul, in my case. Initially she also provided an adrenal tonic and within 3 days I experienced some positive affects! I felt a lot calmer, and not so overwhelmed and breathless. This became an ongoing tonic for some time.

She also confirmed that I suffered with sluggish bowels (Irritable bowel) as well as a candida overload in my system, due to these other factors. Over the last 18 months, she has addressed many elements including—parasites, fungal infections, nasal congestion, Vitamin B deficiencies (blood tests), Vitamin D deficiency (blood tests) along with other vitamin and associated deficiencies and liver detoxification processes. Thus, **infections and Nutritional deficiencies** have been 'prime target' through this process.

The Naturopath has identified that for me to feel in good health with increased energy—we need to aim for _sub optimal levels_ (as for many people with FMS)—as the body has been overloaded and over worked (under intense stress whilst struggling to cope) and needs the additional support, to heal and restore 'normal' functioning.

It was also suggested earlier on, that I add to my diet psyllium husks, manuka honey, ginger, garlic and Aloe Vera juice. Manuka Honey, garlic and ginger all have gentle but positive effects of the gut, having many beneficial properties—a couple of these being natural anti biotic and anti-fungal.

I have also struggled with 'SAD's (Seasonal Affective Disorder) through the gloomy months—worsened in last 4 to 5 years. My body seems to need regular sunshine and fresh air. Consequently, 5HTP was added to the list for the winter months and improved my frame of mind and coping ability through the winter.

Originally, although we discussed my current diet and **nutrition**—it was only part of our 'regime'. I had been honest with this naturopath and said that as my energy levels were low, I wouldn't be able to cope with making big changes to what I was eating at that time. I also stated that I would not be able to follow a diet if it was full of the things that I didn't like and/ or wouldn't eat. I have always been a fairly simple, plain eater and therefore she spent considerable time finding what I did like and what I could increase— that was of the 'good influence'.

She gave me simple 'recipes' and ways of incorporating a few new options of the 'better food choices', but within the scope of what I would eat. I knew I wouldn't continue a diet filled with salad and greens and therefore she included things that I like in order to make it sustainable. Of course, she eliminated some things completely—carbohydrates, bread, potatoes, sugar filled and refined foods.

But kept it fairly simple (brown rice with vegetables that I love). I have since also made some changes to Chenoa's diet and she has also experienced positive effects from these changes. Some of the changes were challenging at first, but with the menu guidance, support and planning that was given to me—I now wouldn't look back, as I have experienced an alternative and no longer miss those things—although I loved them (for example white bread)!

I made a very enlightened discovery—linked to long term weight management and healthy nutrition. That is, *it's not so much about what you 'don't' eat AS* <u>*what* **YOU DO** *eat*</u>.

We may diet and reduce or swap certain foods when trying to lose weight or manage weight—but most important is what you DO eat. I never ate badly or excessively but I can now see that what I **was** eating needed to change, as well as increase. My body needed more of the good stuff! It needed more of the good stuff, due to its poorly functioning state.

It's the good stuff that ensures the balance is right to reduce the bad stuff (candida etc). Optimal function means elimination of infections, parasites, fungae—as well as good nutritional intake to assist the natural balance. Before we can restore (via improved diet), we need to attempt to address the nutritional deficiencies and underlying problems.

Bit by bit, and piece by piece I have made continual progress forwards (under the care of my Naturopath), and again I have learnt and continue to learn so much in this area. I still experience positive change(s) (as far as I am willing to continue to make dietary changes)—with the intention of totally restoring and replenishing my health. I have learnt so much about diet and more importantly, have become an avid follower of the field of 'nutritional medicine'. Initially, I pressed forward and persevered with the thinking that 'it's not going to do any harm'. But, now my thinking has shifted to 'my body deserves to have this care and nutrition'. Along with the positive outcomes I know (experience) and feel.

And what great role modelling our daughter is having from just this part of the journey alone! Multi-dimensional effects and still I move forward, learn, implement and make changes to habits that have been quite ingrained. I have learned to respect and never underestimate the importance of good nutrition and diet, the digestive processes and the Gut!

I strongly urge anyone else with health issues to consider learning more (in this regard) and undertaking juicing and a real effort to make some changes—you won't regret the effort! Even if the effort is dedicated only for a few weeks (or month)— it will be worth it and your body will heed some beneficial results.

***Illness is an opportunity for awareness and freedom.***

## 3/ PHYSIOTHERAPIST

Originally I sought the services of physio for obvious reasons related to the physical pain that had been surfacing. More specifically, the extremely tender spots on each thigh—which were deemed 'bursitis' early in the piece. My visits continued, as the pain increased. The physio treated my neck, shoulders, back and was becoming concerned about my increasing unexplained pain together with my rapidly declining energy levels and deteriorating health. The physio didn't doubt my pain levels, but at the same time he couldn't work out why the problems kept recurring without relief.

He witnessed my increasingly pale complexion, and was concerned about my exhaustion and fatigue. At this time other tests were being conducted with my GP, in search of answers. I was also awaiting the consultation with the Rheumatologist Specialist, and this physio was aware of this.

At one point the physiotherapist suggested acupuncture, with the desired outcome of increasing energy levels. Initially he tried this in very low key fashion and it made me feel slightly unwell, but I decided to have a second treatment at my next visit.

After the second treatment I couldn't even stand up. At the conclusion of the treatment I felt a little weird in the head, 'spaced out', dizzy, unusual. After a recovery time (to sit up) and some water, I was able to stand and headed out to reception area. However, once there I felt overcome with dizziness, and nausea. I had to lie down and didn't know if I was going to vomit.

I had to lie across a few chairs out in the waiting area for around half an hour, and still couldn't sit up. I knew I just wanted to get to bed as I felt so unwell but knew I wasn't going to be able to drive home or anywhere. I had to get the receptionist to call someone for me—to come and pick me up. Once home, I had to go to bed and didn't get out of bed for over 24 hours. I still felt unwell for a couple of days and we never did that again!

The Physiotherapist called our home, after around an hour—to see how I was. He didn't really understand what had happened, but it obviously had a negative effect on my system (including lowering my blood pressure even further). This certainly indicated to the physio that there were certainly some issues being challenged within my body!

At my next visit he was extremely cautious and we decided that all we would do was treat the pain, for the short term. He informed me that until we had more results back from blood tests (and until I had spoken with the doctors) and until we knew what was going on within my physical system—that we would only treat pain as best we could. No more acupuncture of any other interventions until more clarity was obtained!

As I became aware that I had to try to find my own ways of managing the pain and given the physio had provided some useful strategies and techniques, I stopped physio appointments. He also thought it best, until we knew what the doctors wished to do.

Once I received the diagnosis of FMS, I did again seek another physio—to now move forward with appropriate gentle movement and exercises. I relied again on word of mouth and connected with a physio that was more 'specialised' in FMS. This physio was female, and initially showed me useful stretches and exercises I could do at home to keep my muscles 'working' and to avoid more problems from lack of use. She also gave me exercises to assist with pain management. I did do these exercises and felt confident with this physiotherapist. Again, after a few visits and with increased confidence I didn't feel the need to continue the regular visits, unless the need arose. But, I now had an appropriate physio that I could go back to and consult with at any time.

I did require her services again—due to tennis elbow which flared up. This added to the mix for a short while and produced more pain along with its own set of challenges. As if grocery shopping and lifting wasn't enough of a challenge!

I also sought her input again earlier last year (2011), after being thrown off a horse! Now that was really spectacular—but incredibly painful at the time. It also again put an abrupt halt to my increasing exercise regime (home treadmill).

From my best intentions, for our 'horse crazy' daughters 10th birthday wish—I sustained injury that ensured I kept low profile AGAIN for around 6 weeks! Chenoa had expressed a wish—her and I undertaking a trail ride on horseback. However, my horse had quite different ideas . . . He jumped, kicked and bucked—and I actually managed to stay on! But, then he realised just that fact—I was still there—so, off he went again—with a tremendous buck and reared up—until I lost consciousness and next thing I remember I was laying on the ground—flat on my back! The following weeks were not pretty and were very uncomfortable indeed and recovery took several weeks. But, looking back this situation could have been far worse! I was indeed very lucky. Although, darling daughter knows not to expect me to do the horse riding thing again anytime soon!

So, for people with FMS I suggest you link in with a well informed and knowledgeable physiotherapist as you will require their support from time to time. It's good to know that you have one that is aware of your 'story' and has your history and records—and when things are not going so well, you can seek their valuable input. Many physiotherapists also offer aqua aerobics classes (which I have done) and Pilates (which I have also done) as part of their practice. Both of these can be of great benefit to anyone, but especially to people with FMS.

***The present moment is your point of power.***

## 4/ MASSAGE

For around the last 6 years I have treated myself to regular gentle therapeutic massage. As it is covered under my Private Health Insurance, the cost has been minimal when weighing up the benefits on the body as well as a form of relaxation. From 2007 through until quite recently I tried to schedule in an hour massage every month. The benefits from massage are very well documented and I would highly recommend this treatment for people with FMS, even if it's less frequent. However, you need to ensure its 'gentle' and the massage therapist has some knowledge and understanding of FMS. I have accessed some massages that have been convenient BUT they have been far too heavy handed, and left me sore for quite a while. It's not very enjoyable to experience at the time, nor the after affects!

Massage is very beneficial for eliminating toxins and, therefore, ensure plenty of water is put into your system before and after the massage. It also works well to have the massage later in the day and preferably on a day where physical labour is minimal and will also be minimal the following day! I used to go straight from work, at 7pm and by the time I got home I would be quite relaxed and try to stay that way and head off to bed as soon as possible (9pm).

Also, try not to be deterred if some side effects are experienced in the early days of those first massages. Due to the stimulation and 'detox' affect, I often used to get little colds or minor illness—that I am sure were after effects of stirring things up. However, after you have been a few times then this should settle.

Ensure you inform the therapist of any discomfort or ailments upon your next visit. A good therapist will be able to fully support you and your needs, in relation to your condition (FMS). Also remember that people with FMS must have very little pressure applied and gentle massage(s)—eg 'therapeutic massage' or the experience will be negative and uncomfortable due to pain.

**The challenge of life is to overcome.**

## 5/ KINESIOLOGY

This form of treatment is a little less known but also aligns within the scope of Natural Therapies—eg many people have not heard of it and a few asked me 'what is kinesiology?'. It may not suit everyone. I was drawn to try this at a time when I was open minded; seeking answers and had nothing to lose. I sought a fully qualified Practitioner who was registered and therefore I was able to claim for the treatment through my Private Health Insurance. So, again, the outlay cost to me was minimal.

I was visiting approx. once a month. I would like to add here that when going through initial stages of FMS, one feels like all one does is attend Doctor's appointments, undertake medical 'duties'—blood tests etc. Whilst this is a gruelling time filled with uncertainty, I found that some of these 'complementary' treatments provided a sense of balance. It was also another person to talk to, and who would listen to how impacts were affecting lifestyle. These therapists provided another perspective and I found this kept my hope alive. I continued to hope that I would restore some of my health and that my energy and lifestyle may return. I had to remain optimistic.

I was first made aware of Kinesiology through an information session for parents of children with Autism. This Practitioner (Robyn) truly believed in what she did and spoke about the benefits and improvements she had witnessed in this area of Autism. I also knew of another person who was accessing this treatment from Robyn, and recommended Robyn, as they were of the opinion that these methods had been useful and beneficial for them. I figured, if the cost was minimal and even if the positive effects are 'in the mind', then it was still far better than taking endless medications that were impacting on the body—as well as the pocket. Private Health Insurances have also come a long way in recognising a wider range of treatment options, for improved wellbeing of their consumers.

The idea of Kinesiology is that any imbalance of physique, chemistry, nutrition or emotion can be detected by the variation of stress resistance in various muscle groups. The practitioner can then treat what he or she finds by employing methods of acupressure on certain points of the anatomy and this readjusts the nervous system. The muscles become monitors of stress and imbalance within the body where 'Muscle Testing', the key technique in Kinesiology, is used as an effective and versatile tool for detecting and correcting various imbalances in the body which may relate to stress, nutrition, learning problems, and injuries and so on.

Holistic kinesiology aims to improve your health and wellbeing by stimulating your body's own healing potential. It works on the principle that the body, mind and spirit are connected and through the balance of these, full health can be achieved. Kinesiology sessions may include counselling, acupressure, colour therapy, sound therapy, reflexology, emotional release techniques, chakra and meridian balancing, flower essences, homeopathy and nutritional changes.

Kinesiology may be used to assist with—learning difficulties, brain function, pain relief, insomnia, depression, relationship problems, hormonal disorders, structural problems (back aches), addictions, fear and phobias and a variety of other conditions.

The proof to me was in the first couple of visits, where Robyn identified some of my issues—without prior knowledge—via the techniques that are used by Kinesiology Practitioners.

I attended approx. 10 visits with Robyn, and as well as the treatment I also enjoyed some lovely chats with her. She was a beautiful soul, very gentle, kind and caring and again I considered myself grateful that she had crossed my path and come into my life at that part of this journey. I have no regrets about this treatment for me—as our many chats also assisted me emotionally and psychologically. Robyn was also counsellor to many—who were on a path to seek out ways to help them cope with whatever they were there for. This aspect was just as important and beneficial as the treatment.

The only reason why I discontinued this type of treatment was that my appointments got cancelled and I was informed that this was necessary due to ill health. I did not seek out another Kinesiologist, as Robyn had come into my life very easily and I was apprehensive about seeing another Practitioner. Although Robyn did resume her practice at a later date (approx. 12 months later) I did not feel the same need any more for that particular type of treatment. For me, this treatment was short term and I had then found useful alternatives.

If Kinesiology is something you may like to investigate further, I would strongly suggest the best way is via 'word of mouth' as recommendation is the best referral source. You do not need a referral from your doctor for initial consult—nor does your doctor need to be aware or informed of your intent to consult a Kinesiologist. However, in my case Robyn knew my GP through her own networks. My GP had great respect for her and he remained open minded to this type of treatment—or never suggested otherwise. Therefore, (as far as I am aware) he didn't have any concerns about my visits/appointments. I also suggest that prior to initial consultation you do contact your Private Health Insurer, and check both your eligibility status, as well as if the Practitioner/therapist is accredited and registered with the Insurer as a Service Provider.

Unfortunately for many, Robyn passed away in September 2011 at the age of 46 years. This was extremely sad, as we all felt very lucky to have had her in our lives. Her Professional service, as well as her beautiful nature and care and compassion are all very sad losses to many individuals—as well as to this world.

May you Rest In Peace beautiful Robyn . . . .

*Remind yourself of all the things you are grateful for.*

## 6/ PSYCHOLOGIST

Originally I was able to access some psychology sessions via workplace counselling. However, as this was limited I also knew I could continue to access this support via the 'Access to Mental Health Care Plan', under Medicare and via GP referral. My GP was open to this when I suggested this to him, late in 2008 when we discussed 'how I wanted to progress from that point'.

He provided the documentation that I needed, and I was able to continue with the same psychologist and receive the Medicare payment and this was bulk billed through Medicare. Provided my visits were monthly, I was able to continue under this scheme for approx. 12 months.

This intervention provided me acceptance and emotional support immediately. It enabled me to discuss my concerns and have them validated without being judged. However, it was more beneficial than counselling may have been due to the interventions that were used and possibly more affective. That is not to say anything negative about counselling, however, the mindfulness techniques and more concrete strategies and interventions were what assisted me greatly at that time.

The psychologist acknowledged my experiences and I was able to verbalise my concerns without feeling like a hypochondriac. Due to a limited support network and lack of understanding and awareness of FMS, the validation I received helped me to 'normalise' my feelings and concerns.

I always felt better after the sessions and went away with things to ponder, and next session we would pick up where we left off. I was able to feel and express my sadness, confusion and grief in a constructive way. It was ME time and I was free to cry, to express myself but before I left each session was also given something positive and helpful.

Early in my visits, the psychologist knew that my biggest issue of challenge was around sleep and why I couldn't sleep. I was directed to what is called MINDFULNESS and is a way of accepting thoughts and feelings and acknowledging them BUT NOT buying into them. Thus, reducing anxiety and changing way of thinking about them. I was given a CD and provided with an author (and suggested books), who also developed this CD. I listened to the CD at night, and if I woke through the night and have trouble getting back to sleep. It was a simple way to refocus thoughts and it assisted greatly.

We also worked through various work related issues and looked at what other strategies and resources would be useful for me. It was very beneficial to have someone 'on my side', and was given back my power, in a situation where I felt I had lost all power and control.

These sessions were emotionally supportive but the use of practical supports and resources were also included. One of the good and helpful books I read at that time was 'The Happiness Trap' (Russ Harris). I was guided in a practical way to address certain problems and issues in a systematic and logical way. I was given tools that I was able to further develop after the sessions ceased.

The sessions encouraged and assisted me with my communication about what was happening for me, and the results and benefits for me were amazing—for such a short time each month. They were at times tiring and emotional, but this is what also assists our healing processes.

I would highly recommend this type of support, as it increases our valuable skills base for long term use in our lives. It also provided immediate relief and support. I would not hesitate in any way in seeking this psychologist out again, in the future if the need arose!

## EXERCISE

Exercise was another vital aspect in my long term management. I was the one primarily responsible for this area of contribution. Earlier in the illness, I relied on gentle stretching and limbering movements (pilates and yoga) and then slowly moved 'up' to steady walking.

In early 2010 I borrowed a treadmill from another family member for approx. 3 months and then we purchased our own. We just looked for a very basic walking treadmill, of relatively minimal cost. I was not out to work towards intensive work outs or run marathons. Thus, the cost was only minimal (from the wonderful Big W Department store)! It was hoped this would increase energy, assist with stress, increase muscle tone, bone strength and stamina whilst also assisting weight management.

Initially the pace was slow, and the timeframe short. I chose not to select any incline and left the machine on flat terrain. As per what I had learned about 'pacing' and not over doing things, I began cautiously.

Even now, I find I rarely feel like doing the walking time, but know that I need to make this effort. How I feel fluctuates daily and I modify my time and pace electronically on the machine, accordingly. I still find that the first 5 minutes are challenging. Then I don't think I will make it past the 10 minute mark. The period of 10 to 13 minutes is most challenging for me. Now, after 2 years of consistent effort—I am finding that once I get to 15 minutes, then it becomes easier and my body 'wants' to keep going. Persistence is one of the vital keys!

Even if I only go very slowly, I try very hard to get past 15 minutes. The beauty of these machines is that we can do this, and also track the time, calories burnt and distance quite accurately. I also prefer the convenience of being able to do this at any time, which makes it easier to jump on—than if I had to get changed, and go out for a walk. It's also great when the weather is not good—as the walking can still be done. Even with children doing homework, or sick—no need to leave the house! Mine is also outdoors (under cover) and I enjoy looking out over the yard, watching birds in the trees and crank up the music on my Ipod, when I need some motivation. It is good ME time. More time to keep topping up on positive thoughts and practise optimistic thinking!

I have been known to do two lots of 10 minutes on days I really struggled with energy and not feeling too great, and this flexibility comes with treadmills. It all adds up, and recently I managed to get up to 30 mins, a couple of times a week, at a fairly fast pace (and another 2 or 3 days of 20 mins). No marathons yet, but definite improvement.

There were frustrating times along the way. Many times, I would make some improvements, only to CRASH. Then it would take time to rebuild this confidence again as well as the inclination! So, often it's 3 steps forward and 5 steps backwards, but feels much, much worse at the time—if we allow the negative thoughts to grow! Then there were times when obviously it stressed my body and after moving forward, would then have an episode of acute illness or swine flu etc. The important thing was to take the time off again, allow the body to recover BUT not wait for too long before starting again.

I wouldn't go so far to say as it will help me with weight loss yet, as I don't go fast enough or often enough to burn too much fat. BUT, it definitely assists with **weight management** and must be good for metabolism.

It just takes time, patience, and dedicated commitment. Don't give up even when it seems hopeless!

**_Negative emotion comes from feeling disempowered._**

**_Empowerment leads to positive emotion._**

## Chapter Two

*'Do what you can*
*With what you have*
*Where you are'*
*(Theodore Roosevelt).*

# Resources
# And Strategies

I must admit that by nature, I was not a 'naturally' optimistic person. Due to my previous experiences and earlier years, it was easy for me to succumb to negative thoughts when faced with difficult situations, people, challenges and experiences.

However, I discovered in my 'depth of despair' that the one and only person that held responsibility for taking control of how I was thinking . . . WAS ME! No matter what happened, what choices I made—**'if it's to be—it's up to me'.**

Unfortunately, although many others knew things just weren't right—they held back. It was also very hard for me initially to explain what was happening, as there was so much uncertainty and what I did know, I found too hard to explain as people 'didn't understand'. So, partly for a while I chose to shut them out, due to fear and uncertainty—it was easier and took less energy.

However, I also quickly discovered that the phone stopped ringing, and the questions quickly ceased and there were not many knocks at the front door. People got on with their own lives—whether or not mine was on hold. People's lives are busy, and their lifestyles hectic. But, again I realised instead of being bitter, angry or hurt—that I just had to look for my own strength and get on with IT. But, first I had to work out what IT actually was! Although I had historically been a very sociable person, who mixed well, had many friends, colleagues and acquaintances—I had also come to enjoy my own company from time to time.

So, I had to take responsibility, take realistic action by adopting my own way of coping. I had to remain open to learning and open to changing what needed to be changed—or at least give new things a go and see how they go.

For me, I chose to trek down the inspirational, uplifting pathway and see where it led me and how affective it may be! Just perhaps by changing my thoughts to positive thoughts and by trying to become more optimistic I may improve my wellbeing.

I had always been an independent, creative and resourceful (often from necessity) person and I found that there were many things that could be used and tried—but, I could also still remain private about my own issues. I didn't need to tell everyone around me about FMS—as it wasn't going to be any more productive.

In some ways, I avoided talking about it (FMS and/or my health) at all for some time. Even to this day, until this book appeared, most people around me have not been aware of what really has transpired for our family. I don't intend for anyone to feel guilty but I didn't feel that it would assist me with the process of changing to more optimistic thought. Just because we talk about it with others doesn't always bring good results—if the others involved don't have any awareness or understanding about FMS. Whilst it is important to raise awareness and understanding of FMS, we do this more affectively when we have more energy, understanding and competence within our own situation.

Whilst we need to seek support and have people to confide in, talk to and use as sounding board—we need to select these people wisely. They need to be people who will make us feel better after talking with them about it. Rather than making us feel more negative, hopeless, uncertain, frustrated or even guilty (often unknowingly).

I chose to surround myself with positive people, read inspiring books, used positive affirmations, listened to positive music. (I also cried when I needed to and expressed frustration and annoyance when I needed to—but with the appropriate support to ensure this time to also be used in the best possible way).

Optimism is a school of thought (philosophy) based on believing that life is great. That—in the long run, good will win over bad. No matter what happens to us, how many problems or challenges that we confront—there is always some good. It's a decision made to look on the bright or positive side of life. I still work hard on this every day, and sometimes I am not so good—but, mostly once I am over my 'over reacting' (sometimes meltdowns!) then I will move into better thoughts about whatever situation has presented.

## The Optimist Creed.

*To be so strong that nothing can disturb your peace of mind.*

*To talk health, happiness and prosperity to every one you meet.*

*To make all your friends feel that there is something in them.*

*To look at the sunny side of everything and make your optimism come true.*

*To think only of the best, to work only for the best and to expect only the best.*

*To be just as enthusiastic about the success of others as you are about your own.*

*To forget the mistakes of the past and press on to the greater achievements of the future.*

*To wear a cheerful countenance at all times and give every living creature you meet a smile.*

*To give so much time to the improvement of yourself that you have no time to criticise others.*

*To be too large for worry, too noble for anger, too strong for fear, and too happy to permit the presence of trouble.*

## FACEBOOK

Another useful tool that enabled access to inspiration and positive thinking over the last 2 years (when I FINALLY joined), is the wonderful Facebook!

I say wonderful, as it is—when used appropriately and its full benefits are tapped into safely and with awareness. It is also especially valuable when a person is housebound. Facebook can become a good 'positive' connection and can prevent or minimise social isolation. Throughout the day it is one way of easy, effortless company without demands. It can also have negative impacts and must be used cautiously, as many 'friends' may use as a platform to express their frustrations and negativity and/or it can become of competitive nature for those seeking social 'status' amongst their peers.

However, the individual potentially chooses what the purpose of facebook may be—for the individual themselves. For example, I 'liked' pages that were useful, uplifting, inspirational and cheerful. That means I would then receive positive quotes and enlightening information to scroll through and read regularly. Again the more positive is the content we have coming through to read, the more uplifted we can keep our mind and thinking. Some examples of these useful pages—'This Too Shall Pass', 'Positively Positive', 'We are here to inspire', Doreen Virtue Official fan Page, 'Spiritual Bliss', 'Wake Up Women', 'Star Light', Hay House, '12 Steps to Self Empowerment', 'Wisdom Quotes', 'You Are Enough', 'The Social Butterfly' just to name a few. There are also pages that specifically relate to Fibromyalgia if this is also of personal interest.

A combination and mixture of pages is best, and also through facebook, access is widely available to support groups, and interest groups. I have now linked in with a support group, as well as a food/ nutrition group as well as a few others. This ensures connection and discussion with other like-minded people, who may be able to offer support, guidance, reassurance and useful strategies. These pages and groups can also stimulate discussion and provide challenge to ones thinking in a thought provoking manner. Again, in my case I chose a variety and thus balance. I also didn't just focus on FMS, I also went wider in regards to other chronic illnesses and indeed even terminal illness.

I hold the belief that we are all the same, deep inside. If we strip away our outer layer (of challenge and life experiences), below this we are all sharing the same feelings—frustration, grief, sadness, disappointment etc. As well, on the flip side we may go through different experiences but encounter many similarities AND many of us are just trying to link together and network for the benefit of all. Many of us share the same desired outcome; which is—to spread some positivity and attempt to lift people beyond their current challenge or situation or drama.

The writing of this book also prompted me to create a facebook page entitled 'Fibromyalgia Wellbeing', with the aim that through this page I may link in with, and empower others along a similar path. The page I created follows the same philosophy as this book—in that I believe true wellbeing will occur with a combination of approaches utilised that respect and nurture our physical—psychological—spiritual elements. Thus the page provides not only links with information and useful articles about the condition, but also brings in thought provoking ideas that hopefully challenge the thinking/habits of the individual whilst also respectful (and encouraging) of spiritual health. It refrains from strict definition(s) of spirituality as well as denominational beliefs.

I have connected with a select few people on a more personal level, through this facebook platform. I am sure that the people that run these pages have also learned about Fibromyalgia through my posts and hopefully we help each other in our learning! A couple of near and dear stand outs in this regard are people that WANT to respect our condition, and learn about it, and they communicate and respond to my page and comments in an open minded and non-judgemental way.

One shining example of one of these beautiful people (and another wonderful Facebook page), is

Ros who has created a community and page entitled *'FindingUrWings'*. Ros has unknowingly provided some much needed inspiration and lifted me up on many days. I have utmost respect for her and as well as being reflective of LOVE, she also has the most amazing story! She shines her light and is very authentic in all her actions. Ros shares her own personal journey through her life experiences, learning, spiritual growth and healing. Her spiritual transformation took place (with gusto) in 2006 when she attended a life changing workshop. A workshop that made her look deep within her heart, and challenged her to peel back the layers of the onion—and she was never the same again! Ros states openly that her transformation continues every day.

Ros' Facebook page (**Findingurwings**) was created after her diagnosis of stage 3 breast cancer, mastectomy, chemotherapy, radiation therapy and Herceptin treatments. Ros believes that many roads are shown to us at different times of our life. She also believes that cancer is a WORD and not a sentence. She encourages people when challenged—to try to see that 'anything is possible and all things can change'—rather than choosing fear. Ros' biggest message for us is to LOVE YOURSELF UNCONDITIONALLY', and look within!! She is one amazing, special, unique, beautiful and inspiring lady and I feel privileged to be sharing stories and working towards similar outcomes, albeit along different pathways! (I have information about how to connect with Ros, in the resources section at the end of this book.)

Another wonderful facebook page is entitled 'De-Stress And Be Happy', and is managed by the wonderful Kerry. Basically, in a nutshell, Kerry believes that 'together we can create the optimum health and wellbeing that you have been searching for'. Kerry draws on personal and Professional knowledge that guides and underpins her facebook page. Kerry discovered that there was a lack of creative, positive, common sense information regarding proactively looking after your physical, emotional and mental health and wellbeing. Her idea is to ENABLE people to help themselves. To support people in the process of obtaining the understanding, that THEY can positively influence their own health and wellbeing.

Kerry encourages people to take ownership for their current situation—and to then move forward by choosing to create (for themselves) a new, empowering, stronger and supportive personal reality. Kerry imparts this message in a nonthreatening, no blame, forward thinking environment, which potentially could benefit as many people as possible. Her facebook page    www.facebook.com/de.stressandbehappy provides a forum to share information and gain knowledge in a positive environment. (Information about how to contact Kerry is also contained in the Resource section.)

As these pages strongly mirror my own intentions, and reflect similar desired outcomes, I have come to know these 2 ladies on a more personal level.

I encourage you to check them out, along your own journey. You will only have positivity to be gained—from the very best of intentions—from some of the best people you may ever meet!

## MUSIC

Music is something we all have our own preference which is personal to us and influenced by many factors.

I have an avid passion about social justice, community, fairness and advocacy for those less fortunate. This has been reflected through my career choices, my studies (TAFE and University), as well as my keen participation for nearly 20 years in voluntary community work—often alongside paid work. Participating and contributing to community is very important to me and something I believe in. I believe that we all have strengths and the capacity to add something to our community. We all have our own unique strengths and value(s), and we may contribute in many ways. Sometimes, it can be the little things that we can contribute that have the capacity to make the biggest impact on others.

Therefore, for many years one of my favourite songs that holds significant meaning and importance is that of Pink Floyd = *'On the Turning Away'*. I can listen to this every day and never tire of it. I relate to it, and the message portrayed. Therefore—I just love it. This is my choice—another person may not connect with it at all.

*'On the turning away from the pale and downtrodden, and the words they say which we won't understand . . . Don't accept that what's happening, is just a case of all the suffering—or you'll find that your joining in . . . the turning away.*

*It's a sin that's somehow, light is changing to shadow, and casting a shroud over all we have known . . . . etc etc . . . . On the wings of the night, as the daytime is slurring, where the speechless unite in a silent accord, using words you will find it strange—mesmerised as they light the flame, feel the new winds of change . . . on the wings of the night.*

*No more turning away, from the weak and the weary . . . No more turning away from the coldness inside, just a world that we all must share . . . It's not enough just to stand and stare. Is it only a dream that there will be no more turning away?'*

Some people like classical music, others like Jazz. For me, especially over the last 5 to 6 years—I have turned to peaceful, calming, inspirational and even slightly spiritual music. There has been some music that I can listen to any time of the day and I can appreciate the depth, and connect with it. It gives me strength and the words hold true meaning. It makes feel peaceful, grounded, relaxed and even stronger in my SELF. This can only be positive!

One of my favourite and most significant songs related to FMS and my journey is Miley Cyrus 'The Climb'.

*'Every step I'm taking, every move I make feels lost with no direction . . . my faith is shaken', but I . . . gotta keep tryin', gotta keep my head held high.*

*Theres always gonna be another mountain, I'm always gonna want to make it move . . . always gonna be an uphill battle, sometimes I'm gonna have to lose . . . ain't about how fast I get there, ain't about whats waiting on the other side . . . it's the climb.*

*The struggles I'm facing, the chances I'm taking, sometimes might knock me down but . . . know I'm not breaking . . . I may not know it, but these are the moments that I'm gonna remember most yeah, just gotta keep going and I . . . I gotta be strong, just keep pushing on . . . .'*

I also get great strength from The Pretenders 'Forever Young', as it refers to strong foundations and enduring change.

*'May you always do for others and let others do for you ... May you build a ladder to the stars, and climb on every rung ... May you stay Forever Young.*

*May you grow up to be righteous, may you grow up to be true, may you always know the truth and see the light surrounding you.*

*May you always be courageous, stand upright and be a star ... May you stay ... Forever Young.*

*May your hands always be busy, may your feet always be swift, may you have a strong foundation when the winds of changes shift. May your heart always be joyful, may your song always be sung ... may you stay ... Forever Young'.*

Macy Gray's 'Beauty in the World' is also full of hope.

*'I know your fed up, life don't let up—for us ... all they talk about is whats been going down and whats been messed up—for us ... when I look around, I see blue skies, I see butterflies for us—listen to the sound, and lose it in sweet music, and dance with me ... 'Cos theres beauty in the world, so much beauty in the world—always beauty in the world, so much beauty in the world, so shake your booty boys and girls,*

*for the beauty in the world, pick your diamond, pick your pearl, there is beauty in the world.*

*. . . . Notice the blue skies, notice the butterflies—notice me . . . stop and smell the flowers, and lose it in sweet music and dance with me, 'Cos there is beauty in the world . . . .*

*. . . . When you don't know what you to do, don't know if you'll make it through—remember God he's given you—beauty in the world—so love, . . . yeah love . . . There is beauty in the world'.*

BLISS is another amazing artist with a beautiful voice, and I still enjoy listening to (calming and spiritual) 'A Hundred Thousand Angels' album, as well as 'YOU'. Jade Ambroze (a fellow South Australian) has been uplifting and bright and I also enjoy Olivia Newton Johns more recent peaceful and calming CD's.

These artists and specific songs I have listened to very regularly. Whenever I feel a little in need of a lift—I still look for them! Many of these songs are also part of my almost daily listening regime.

You will find your own sources of connection, but great results can be achieved by keeping the songs positive and with meaningful lyrics. I had them firstly on CD's. I had a portable CD player (single/small) and ear phones. I would listen when walking, when lying down (resting), and even through the night when I couldn't sleep.

I have since downloaded onto my Ipod and use in much the same way. I find it helpful to listen to the peaceful music as I relax to go to sleep.

Basically, when you are trying to relax and find your anxiety is high and thoughts are running riot in your mind and you can't switch off—an easy strategy is to listen to the positive music. It changes the focus and calms the thoughts.

## BOOKS

I acknowledge that many people with FMS do not have the concentration span or the energy to read for long periods of time. I also acknowledge that I have had an avid love of reading, as well as a passion and interest in peoples' stories and their histories. I am fascinated by hearing stories, especially those filled with strength, adversity and determination. These again are the most positive and enriching stories to read at this time. As I needed to be selective about what I read (due to making it count, lack of energy) I had to ensure that I read books that had positive affect on my wellbeing.

I read a lot of information that was clinically based and also craved the knowledge of FMS. However, this required balance with positive reading experiences. Even if I only had 15 minutes of opportunity to read, I could make a positive difference by reading something enlightening and enriching. It is also another useful and positive way to stop or minimise negative thinking.

At my worst time, I read an article in a women's magazine about a truly amazing woman—Tania Hayes. Tania wrote and amazing and inspirational love story about her journey as a Carer for her husband, Warren. This book is entitled **'Love Has No Limits'.** I purchased this book and this was the start of my passion for this inspirational reading. I got so engrossed in this book, and thoroughly loved it! It made me smile, it made me feel sadness and grief and it made me see my challenges in the right perspective.

I had the pleasure of meeting Tania and Warren in a Professional capacity, around 9 months later, and I am sure these two people were meant to cross my path—to be a part of my journey. We have remained in contact now for nearly 4 years and I am extremely grateful to have these two people in my life. Tania's book (of their story) was one of the most inspirational and uplifting resources that I could ever have hoped to find at a difficult time.

Tania has continued to inspire me, with her approach to life and her beautiful spirit. We have connected on many levels and she provides me with motivation and strength. They are truly beautiful people who continue to have influence on me to this day! She was, in fact the very first person I discussed the possibility of my own book with. She has mentored me in many different ways, and I hope to remain connected with these people for a long time. These are the type of people I talk of, when I also refer to 'surrounding yourself with positive people'.

Although people like Tania and Warren are unique, and many of us would never actually meet such a calibre of people—we do have many opportunities to create such relationships. We do get opportunities (although rare) to meet such wonderful people. We just need to remain open minded and look for (seek out) these opportunities. When we do we need to be grateful when we have such encounters. We do choose which relationships we nurture and which relationships we need to maintain a healthy distance with.

I read widely after that book, and it's amazing how many positive, inspirational books you can actually find when you seek them and look hard enough!

I found a lot of books written by people who had faced adversity and challenge and became fascinated with how they got through whilst also continuing to move forward in their life. There were many common threads, and this provided me with insight, motivation and perspective to deal with my own issues and challenges.

I really enjoyed many books but the following titles are those I found most heart-warming and helpful—

'The last Lecture' by Randy Pausch

'Tuesdays with Morrie' and others by Mitch Albom

'Never Say Die' by a Great Australian; Chris O'Brien

'Why Me?; Kicking Cancer—and other life changing stuff' by Yvonne Chamberlain

'Lucky Man—Michael J Fox Memoir' and 'Always looking Up—the adventures of an incurable optimist' BOTH by Michael J Fox

'True Colours; Lauren Huxley and her Family ; from Tragedy to Triumph' by Lisa Davies

I will provide another list at the end of this book and include other book titles that I enjoyed greatly.

I also referred often to quick little 'pick me up' titles including—

'The Book for People Who Do too Much' by Bradley Trevor Greive

'Everyday Positive Thinking' and other titles by Louise Hay

'Life is Short . . . Wear Your Party Pants—10 simple Truths that lead to an amazing Life' by Loretta LaRoche.

And another 'gem' I found when seeking titles on stress management

'Know Thyself—The Stress Release Programme' by Craig Hassed.

(A more comprehensive list will appear in Appendix 4 'Recommended Books', at the end of this book).

*I wish you comfort on difficult days*
*Smiles when sadness intrudes*
*Rainbows to follow your clouds*
*Laughter to kiss you lips*
*Sunsets to warm your heart*
*Hugs when spirits sag*
*Beauty for your eyes to see*
*Friendships to brighten your being*
*Faith so you can believe*
*Confidence for when you doubt*
*Courage to know yourself*
*Patience to accept the truth*
*Love to complete your life.*

## OUR OWN PIECE OF SERENITY—
### HOLIDAY VAN PURCHASE APRIL 2008.

When Chenoa was young, we had our own little camper van (trailer with 'pop top' and slide out beds—compact and easy to tow). Then, as she got older (pre-school years) we preferred to stay in 'farm stay' environments or budget motels as we usually only went relatively short distances for one or two nights. As Brenton is self-employed we were very limited when it came to holidays and time away from the business. This is made more difficult, as our home is also the business 'office' and therefore the need for some distance and space is regularly needed and vital.

The 'window of opportunity' generally were (and continue to be) weekends, and the 10 days between Christmas and New Year. It's important for Benton's wellbeing that we go away from home for regular short breaks. I used to look into where we would go and undertake the planning, booking etc.

However, when I became unwell, it was even more important that we get away from home. Some people may call it 'running away' but, everybody takes holidays. Some people get to take several through the year, and go away at least once or twice. We didn't always get this same 'simple luxury', and had to try harder to get this break from the home.

I have always headed to the beach in times of intense stress, confusion and times of uncertainty. Unfortunately, we live around 35 to 40 mins away from any beach. Given my exhaustion was very intense for a long time—this wasn't possible when I most needed this time by the water, beach or sea. I was barely able to drive to Tea Tree Plaza Shopping Centre, which is less than 10 mins away, let alone the drive to the beach.

One day (just after my BIG crash in 2007) a friend mentioned that they had a caravan kept at a caravan park, up the River (Murray). We asked a little about it and I began contemplating the benefits of a similar idea for ourselves.

I made enquiries about prices, and this led me over to the Yorke Peninsula and to various places, depending on what was available on the market at that time. I had thought about Victor Harbor (Flerieu Peninsula—approx. 1hour and 40 mins drive), but actually decided against it—as I was really looking for a nice quiet, coastal place near the sea, not too far from home and not too busy. I had thought in my mind that Victor Harbor was very tourist orientated, too windy, too cold (cooler temperatures) and thus wasn't an option worth considering.

However, after a couple of months of following up on this idea—guess where we ended up purchasing our piece of serenity? Yep, Victor Harbor ended up being our new holiday place. So, we went ahead with the purchase and in April 2008, we began using our new van. And, I must add—Victor Harbor has been a great spot for us for various reasons.

No matter what the weather, there is always so much to do in and around Victor. Good variety of food outlets, supermarkets, tourist attractions and the quietness of where our van is located (for the most part!).

In 2008, 2009 and 2010 we travelled to Victor every second weekend whenever possible, and spent considerable time chilling and relaxing—away from the pressures of home. This provided much relief for me, and I spent many hours in that time—at the beach. Time was spent watching out over the sea, enjoying the sounds, smells and peacefulness that come with being sea side. We have enough home comforts in our van, to make it enjoyable.

But, most importantly, we have others around us and we are part of the community that comes with being in caravan parks. We are especially lucky, as our van is located at the rear of the park amongst other like-minded people who enjoy their holiday time on regular basis. The people around us form a smaller community (annual site holders), within the larger culture of the park community.

Chenoa has friends that she has known for the four years we have been going there. She has a group of friends around the same age, and we have come to know these families quite well. Although not to the extent that we feel we need to spend a lot of time together, but well enough that we are all comfortable with our children spending time together. It gives us all piece of mind that all the families in our part of the park, all look out for each other's' children.

We have been able to feel safe and allow our children a sense on independence, whilst they have had company and established firm friendships over time. So, for Chenoa the networks and friendships are naturally occurring, which is good for me as it takes the pressure off of making things happen with friends etc—especially as she is an only child. It has been very convenient and natural and we are very pleased that we made this decision.

We often have group activities and although I sometimes spend time (have a drink etc) with the other mums or families (that she plays with)—I don't feel any pressure to do so. I haven't felt judged by any of them, as its just all flowed along.

Every New Year's Eve we usually have a 'street party' and all get together, and every now and then we have a meal with another family or spend time with them, but if I am not feeling up to it—then I don't go—no questions asked. I have missed a few of the get togethers, due to ill health but these wonderful people have respected my space and our privacy. We know each other well enough that we can trust each other, but not well enough to intimately know details of their 'business'.

Chenoa has shared several Birthdays and parties with children from the park. They ride their bikes around, swim together, play together, go to the playground, build forts and spend time just safely being kids. In fact, Chenoa learnt to ride her bike without training wheels at Victor. She has learnt many new skills and the environment's also provided opportunities for her to increase her confidence and social skills. This group of children have grown from being little children to becoming pre-teens—together.

I am forever grateful, for the opportunities this lifestyle has created for Chenoa. She has been able to spend time with others, as well as her family—in the best possible way.

She has often not wanted to go outside of the park, as she has been enjoying the park life so much!

I am also extremely thankful that Chenoa has been accepted into the other families. This lifestyle has had a positive influence on all of us, and the friendships have been appreciated. Through all this time, I have not felt judged by others and I appreciate that acceptance more than they may realise.

Although this drive has been a large task on many occasions, it has been worth it. This has kept things simple, and enabled me to spend time in nature, to reflect, to recharge and to provide opportunities for renewal. It has been a great stress management tool and by keeping things simple—has been a very positive step for all members of our family.

The simplicity of the fresh air, listening to and watching the birds, sunsets, watching the water are all part of the reminders of what a vast world we are a part of. It always fills me with awe and wonderment, when coming down the 'Willunga Hill', on our journey home. As South Australian 'locals' would know, this superb lookout view on a clear day reminds me how big and vast just a small portion of the outer Adelaide suburbia is. This 'view' encourages me to keep perspective and reminds me of the **larger than life** life that we are all a tiny part of!

# MOVING TOWARDS WELLNESS (ARTHRITIS SA)—LATE 2008.

In South Australia, the organisation 'Arthritis SA' supports 'Fibromyalgia SA'—who then in turn provide some services and supports to people in SA living with FMS. Their Mission statement is 'To provide information, education, support and encouragement to people living with Fibromyalgia and their families and friends'. I attended several of their Educational Meetings, and also became a member. This membership included subscription for the Fibromyalgia specific newsletter 'Tender Points'. The newsletter(s) kept me up to date with information and some useful strategies and information which were fibromyalgia specific. Through these contacts I came across the 'Moving towards Wellness' course, a self-management course for people with chronic conditions. This course is designed for all people who may be living with, and managing a chronic condition. I was able to attend a course close to home, and for 6 weeks attended a session each week of 2.5 hours.

The cost was relatively minimal, and it provided me with some useful understandings that I was able to implement and become better informed about managing/coping. It was also useful (at that time) to be with other group members and engage in open discussions and sharing—about doctors, about medications, about the highs and the lows. Although the course was not intended as a support group, there were some helpful opportunities to learn from others in similar situations who were struggling with similar issues.

After the course, opportunities were available for joining support groups, which were facilitated via Fibromyalgia SA and available in a variety of locations. However, this was not something I chose to follow up on afterwards—as I was also working and time and energy didn't allow for this support.

For me, I was greatly encouraged to 'keep moving' (in the physical sense) as the importance of this was discussed at length. It was a very valuable course for me and I am again thankful for the timing, as well as the opportunity to attend and benefit from the time spent.

## POSITIVE AFFIRMATIONS (LOUISE HAY).

I have always been a fan of Louise Hay, and have used her resources many times in the past. Over the last 4 years, I began to purchase a few of her books that included positive affirmations. I printed these affirmations off, cut them up and put them up around the home. When I had the opportunity to read, I would include some of these appropriate affirmations in my reading time. But, I also **absorbed** them—not just read them. I wanted to believe in them and they helped me to keep my hope alive.

Using Positive Affirmations was (is) another useful way to change my thinking from worried, anxious and negative into more useful, uplifting and positive. I tried to keep topping myself up with all things positive.

**'My health gets better and better all the time'.**

Louise has many, many uplifting books and has done amazing things over the last 30 years!

I considered Louise's metaphysical explanations of 'dis-ease' in the body, and remained open minded enough to read some of her literature and pondered what she was saying. I do agree with her (and others) and ascribe to her suggestions that we must balance body, mind and spirit for us to be whole and healthy. How we choose to do this is individual to each and every one of us. Whilst I can enlist the support of health Practitioners and doctors, it is MYSELF that needs to decide if I make the choice to be a part of MY healing process. I also figured, if it's positive stuff, then it's certainly not going to do any harm. Healing of Dis-ease needs to become more broadly considered and multi-dimensional. Many levels of healing may need to be embraced and addressed. Healing also occurs from the 'inside'.

According to one of her books FIBROMYALGIA is fear showing up as extreme tension due to stress . . . Interesting!

Pituitary gland = represents the control centre. Very interesting indeed!

And it certainly didn't do me any harm to change my thinking and try to have some faith in life and to trust in myself. I choose to try to make positive changes from **this** day.

I needed to start to take action to balance the body—mind—spirit. Maybe through these actions some healing may then occur.

*Let us rise up and be Thankful*
*For if we didn't learn a lot today, at least*
*we learned a little,*
*And if we didn't learn a little, at least*
*we didn't get sick,*
*And if we got sick, at least we didn't die*
*So let us all be thankful*
*(Buddha).*

# EMPLOYMENT

In May 2007, I changed my place of employment and slightly increased the hours I was working.

The new location was much closer to home, my travel time now only 7 to 8 minutes, instead of 20 minutes. Around 5 months into this new position, I became increasingly unwell.

However, I obviously made a positive impact. At the end of 2007 I received a nomination for 'Employee Recognition Award'! The timing of this was of considerable importance, as it provided further encouragement for what was to be a 'tough road ahead'. I did not win this award, however for me the nomination was very significant and what was important, after being 'new' to this organisation. My immediate colleague was also nominated the same year. However, we were thrilled when this colleague was nominated again the following year, and was a 'joint' winner with another staff person.

Being new into an existing position, I was fortunate enough to be able to work autonomously and mould this position around my planning. Being a 'Typical Type A Over Achiever', we achieved amazing successes and continued to plan a very successful program. Only a few people within my immediate 'team' had been made aware of my health 'restrictions' and struggles.

As I was slowly coming to terms with the fact I was in poor health, I was also dealing with much uncertainty, however I made a pretty major decision. I thought about it long and hard—and I would suggest my decision at this time would not be for everyone. I collected some relevant and concise information about FMS and put it all together and made an appointment with an 'advisor' within the Human Resources Department. I was a little hesitant, as I could have had much to lose by making this bold step. However, I was a little fearful and unsure of the future impacts of my health. I was unsure how this would affect my career in the long term.

I am a person who holds **personal responsibility** very near to my own virtues. I decided that, if I got to the point where I needed help or assistance of any kind—I could not expect this help to come—unless I asked for it. People cannot assist, if they are unaware. I also felt it was important to have this matter recorded on my records, in the event of further deterioration of my health.

The 'advisor' was extremely reassuring and I felt confident that I had done the 'right' thing, for myself and the organisation.

This person assured me of utmost confidentiality and left the door open in the event further support was needed. To this day I have no regrets that I took this very nerve racking step.

At this meeting, we discussed some simple changes that I thought may assist me at least in short term—eg parking closer to front doors of the building, when I needed to load my car in preparation of my group work. Another point of discussion was accessing workplace counselling, with financial support from the organisation. I followed up on these options and I felt a strange sense of relief from being honest and updating them on where things were at for me.

I did access workplace counselling, and then discovered longer term help was available, under 'Access to Mental Health Care Plan' (accessible via GP). Fortunately I spent some time receiving valuable support from a psychologist.

My immediate colleague (and friend) was also kept up to date and was concerned about my health. The support she gave me through this time was invaluable. We had many discussions both formal and informal and I am pretty sure she had her awareness raised, in regards to the issues I was dealing with. She also remained open (and extremely supportive) to any changes I made to the program over the following 18 months—that were intended to benefit the program, but also to better support my work load.

In my down times and when I was in despair, we both recall me saying on more than one occasion 'I am not letting this beat me' . . . 'These health issues are NOT going to win'. I continued to push through and was very determined that my work life would not be affected. I would not go so far as to say that this was an attitude that made my life more difficult. However, it was the attitude (at that time), that helped me to keep going. I knew I needed to continue to work, in a job and role that I loved with the passion that I had—in order to continue getting out of bed in the mornings. It was part of what kept me going and kept me focussed on not giving up. Working with carers helped me to hold onto some perspective, through giving to them through the program—in some ways I was also giving to myself. I was accountable to them, as I was accountable to Brenton and Chenoa and therefore, had to keep putting one foot in front of the other.

Within the role that I had, I was extremely fortunate to have the support of a small group of volunteers. These volunteers greatly assisted me practically through this time. They would meet with me, and help me to do any physical work that needed doing, not to mention the emotional support regarding my work load—in their own way(s).

On the whole, these volunteers were not aware of my health issues and challenges. Except for one 'husband and wife couple' who did have awareness that I wasn't well, and who knew of some of my struggles. They kept this to themselves and continued to ask after my wellbeing and I must admit crying on their shoulder(s) a couple of times. I needed to have some understanding from a couple of people and I greatly appreciate the respect, compassion and understanding that they provided me on personal level—as well as the practical support.

Over time, however, I think it was harder and harder for me to 'hide' when I was struggling, as I became more tired and exhausted in my work. Without the support from these volunteers, I would not have been able to cope for as long as I did.

I am so grateful to them and I feel very lucky to have been in the company (again) of such wonderful warm, caring human beings.

These volunteers were also beside me when I eventually had to inform the participants of the program of my resignation, in March 2011. They supported me to deliver a very difficult message to the wonderful people that had inspired me for so long, in my own journey! Any volunteers are worth their weight in gold but these volunteers were especially endeared to me!

Resigning from my position became necessary due to a combination of factors. I worked within a fairly small team, and we were all very dedicated and focussed on achieving good results for our clients. We were all very busy and under intense pressure. All the team members also had their own lives, with their own challenges and ups and downs—all having their own families.

I could not (and would not) expect the team to carry any extra burden that came from my inability to cope and deliver 100% of the time. I was growing increasingly tired (exhausted!) and became more easily overwhelmed and stressed.

It was too hard to explain to them the impacts resulting from my health. It's hard to explain to others what is very complicated and not well understood. Then there is the energy and time required to explain—of which I had neither!

Also coming into play was my 'accountability' to the larger organisation. Unless I was to make it common knowledge of my health, then I couldn't presume that they would expect anything but the same standard that had existed for 4 years. There were a lot of organisational changes coming into effect thick and fast, and this combined with our already stressful roles, became too much for me to manage—along with managing my health at satisfactory level.

Then there was the client group that I worked with. This group of people have been my inspiration for over 17 years and have added so much richness and depth to my character and my life. I felt that out of respect for them, I needed to acknowledge my time to leave. To pass on the batton to someone who had the energy and passion to continue to deliver to them in the way they deserved. After all, it is not very professional for the group leader to be expecting the group to be supporting her, when the professional role was the other way around. I was very determined not to cross that line. If I could not continue to support them in the way they deserved—then I could not be there. It was not professional for them to support me. It was unprofessional for them to even be aware of my health status! They remained unaware of my ongoing health issues—although I think that a few of them did 'suspect' something.

Some people were surprised when I resigned, however others were not. Over time, I had 'preached' to the client group (carers) that I worked for (with), time and time again—the importance of self-care and seeking help when needed.

I now needed to demonstrate this and practice what I had been 'preaching'.

*Don't mourn for the past*
*Worry about the future*
*Or anticipate troubles*
*But live in the present moment*
*Wisely and earnestly*
*(BUDDHA)*

# SCHOOL

I remember often picking Chenoa up from school in years one and two, and upon getting to her classroom, I used to sit and wait—like the other parents. However, after the children were dismissed, I was still sitting and waiting. Long after everyone else (including parents) had left for the day.

I had to wait for some energy—that would never come, to help us get home. Everyone else had left, but I would wait another 10 mins before heading back to the car.

Some of the other children must have thought this was quite unusual behaviour. I remember on more than one occasion, another child asking me 'why I sat and waited so long, after Chenoa had come out of the classroom'. I simply replied with the truth that I just needed a rest. The only problem was that rest never really helped and I still felt like I dragged my body back to the car. But after getting into the car, we had to get home. Then we had to unpack from school, do homework, prepare tea, and all the other chores that come with that wonderful (said with sarcasm) 'after school time'. The days I did the school pick up after a day at work, were even more painstaking and slow.

This process was further complicated, as it was so difficult to park in close proximity of school, unless one arrived to school at least 20 minutes before the final bell went. This added pressure to my need to leave work on time and get to the school in ample time. If I did not, then I needed to park around 150 metres away from Chenoa's classroom! But, the idea of such a walk was terrifying! However, she was too young not to be collected from her classroom.

Again, I was not one to put my 'burdens' onto others and did not wish to sound like I was complaining, as these matters are not well understood.

After a couple of months passed and my health status continued to deteriorate, I decided to write a letter to the school and request permission to access one of the disability car spaces on the school grounds, right beside the school gate, close to Chenoa's classroom. This was not easy to do, however was necessary at that time. This was complicated because it isn't a simple process with this condition to obtain a 'disability car parking permit'. Thus, being on school grounds, I thought this access to a car park may be an option for me.

Much to my surprise, the school Principal contacted me a couple of days after I sent my letter of request. She discussed and empathised about my situation. She was very open to the possibility of using one of these allocated spaces. She was aware of how many people with correct permits were using the spaces and was confident there were sufficient spaces, to enable me use of one.

She also advised me that she would pass on what we had discussed and decided with the school caretaker, who was on 'duty' after school bell and he monitored these car parks. My car make, colour, registration was given to her—to pass on to the caretaker/groundsman.

So, this strategy worked—I would get there only 5 to 10 mins before the final bell sounded, would access a park and could manage the short walk to the classroom. The caretaker would acknowledge me, and all was well. For a few weeks!

Then, I discovered the 'norm'. Some other parents would (possibly unknowingly) give me the 'glare'. This park was right beside the school access gate and whilst I waited in the car, it didn't 'look good' to others obviously—especially to those parents who knew of me. According to their perception, I had no need to be using this car space. The 'looks' continued and I felt so bad. I decided that unless I approached them individually and told them why I was parking there—then I couldn't continue to park there. So, that was the end of that!

Little did they know that I would be the last person on earth to ever use or access a disability parking space without permission! I am sure I could have gone back to the Principal and worked on another strategy, I just went back to struggling through and having many long waits at the classroom! After a while, the kids did stop asking and just accepted it. It was also useful for those children whose parents would often be late to pick them up—as it gave them someone to wait with!

This situation became a little easier when Chenoa was in year 4 when she was able to have a little more independence. She was more able to find her own way out to the gate after school.

In year 3 (2009), Brenton began assisting by dropping her off to school in the mornings—as even now I struggle most in the mornings. This, at least made the mornings a little easier for me, especially when I went to work from school drop off.

## MEDIC ALERT BRACELET

Due to limited support networks (that were kept informed with my health status and issues) combined with the fact that I was becoming increasingly vague, confused and losing confidence driving—I decided to look into the obtaining one of these bracelets.

I held some concerns, that the episode in 2007 may have been seizure related (and this may happen again). My blood pressure had been low, and I was a little worried that I may faint at some time. If any of these things should happen, then I was able to be cared for appropriately as a result of having this bracelet. It also concerned me that something may occur whilst with my daughter and she was only aged 6 or 7 at that time. I felt she didn't have the knowledge necessary to provide any assistance if needed. It was a little unfair to place her in that position and any such situations 'arise', as it would most likely be frightening enough for her. Whilst she knew I had some health issues, she wasn't fully informed and we limited what we told her due to her age. (She didn't have the capacity to be kept informed and appropriately process and understand). This bracelet was one way to alleviate some of my concerns at that time.

I spoke to my GP, and given this was a personal choice (user pays system), he had no reservations in completing the paperwork with me. I wore the bracelet every day, through my uncertain times and it provided me with great peace of mind.

In 2011, when I received the renewal forms I didn't feel the same need for maintaining/updating the stored information. I found I wasn't wearing the bracelet as much either. This was due to the fact I had stabilised in many areas, and I felt more clear headed and therefore didn't feel so vulnerable. Chenoa is also a little bit older now, and would be better equipped to cope in any such situation.

## STRESS MANAGEMENT THERAPIES

I have been a fan of (Hatha) **yoga** and the benefits of **yoga**—for over 10 years. I participated in yoga before I had Chenoa, as well as whilst pregnant and over the years since then. The stretching and mobility greatly assist people with challenges in these areas. It is also grounding and balancing. It is great for managing stress and a very relaxing and therapeutic technique.

It assisted greatly whilst my mobility was restricted, as I felt it important to keep these muscle's viable and flexible, during the periods of time where my exercise was limited.

The only reason I stopped was that whilst I was working, the night classes became unsuitable and didn't fit in with my family commitments. More recently I have been able to slowly increase my fitness through exercise. Therefore, I do not feel the need is so high for yoga in my life any longer. I would not hesitate to return to yoga at any time, if the need arose. But night classes are still not really an option for me.

I also participated in **Pilates** for approx. 6 months, as well as **aqua aerobics** for a short time. Whilst these are both highly beneficial for many, they were not as enjoyable for me as other techniques have been. For example the whole 'water thing', wearing bathers and dealing with showering, wet bathers etc was too tiring for me. Combined with wet hair, when being self-conscious of very thin hair = not something that made me feel positive and so I avoided this and sought alternatives. I think this is healthy, as often we find out what we DON'T want to engage in, and this prompts us to look further to find what does appeal to each of us as individuals. The important thing is to *try* and continue to *seek.*

I also tried **Tai Chi,** for several months but found this wasn't for me—as I lacked the concentration and coordination at the time. Also contributing to my lack of enjoyment was that the classes that were closest to me and most accessible were in the evening. At that time, I didn't venture out at night time, for various reasons including that dreadful tiresome fatigue. Also by the time I got through that time of afternoon (dinner time etc) I was not good for much let alone driving and getting through such a lesson. Maybe in the future I will have this opportunity again.

I used a variety of **relaxation** and **stress management 'tools'** including incense, candles and aromatherapy. I purchased some nice music, as well as some meditation focussed CD's and listened to these regularly when the need was high. I still love each one of these methods, and 'indulge' in all of them on regular basis—sometimes all at the same time! I also have a very valuable CD with Mindfulness Meditation exercises on it.

I developed a love of Doreen Virtue and remained open to her guidance via faith in angels.

Along with this, I drew comfort from my 'healthy interest' (curiosity) in **Crystal therapy**. I collected many crystals and became intrigued with their properties and their 'benefits'. I learned a great deal and again it was all a positive influence. If nothing else, crystals are relatively cheap to buy, and they are objects of beauty. They look nice and are colourful. They can be grounding and anything that provides that comfort is worth considering. Chenoa has a few of her own, and still uses a couple of them when she has stressful events at school. Eg she carries them in her pocket for comfort when needing to do public speaking or activities that make her anxiety levels peak. There is no harm in any tools that create that affect. Again it is a very personal thing and if it does no harm to anyone else, then it's a positive influence. Better than medication! Remain open to try anything that may be useful to your support.

Around 16 years ago, I did some intensive training for **Reiki**, but due to other distractions haven't kept this up for a long time. However, it is something I have been prompted to consider again in the near future.

As I have also shared, I have great passion for **reading** and this has always been a great hobby from younger years. Another stress management tool I have also actively used is **the beach**—and nowadays I also **walk** whilst there (on regular basis), whenever I can but usually once a week or once a fortnight. (In my least energetic times I couldn't even attempt the 35 minute drive and had this 'beach time' whilst at Victor Harbor, but since leaving my employment 12 months ago I have scheduled this time into 'most' weeks.)

Over the last 10 years I have also enjoyed **scrapbooking** as a creative outlet and hobby. However, whilst in the most intense time with this illness, the desire was there but the energy and creativity was not. Since resigning from my employment, I have rediscovered this hobby and have worked on some pages again. I still have many to do (with photos of Chenoa), and focus intently on this craft for a couple of weeks and then redirect my focus to some other little project. I have done some *little* projects in Chenoa's room, and made some handy and useful modifications (eg jewellery storage etc). It's quite amazing what can be done with paint and some crafty ideas—even on a limited budget. Although I am not a sewing person and have what I call 'limited abilities' when it comes to handicrafts, there are always **creative opportunities** awaiting us. We just need to keep those flames alight!

*Everyone is a house with 4 rooms—a physical, a mental, an emotional and a spiritual. Most of us tend to live in one room most of the time.*

*But, unless we go into every room, every day, even if only to keep it aired—we are not a complete person. (–Indian Proverb.)*

## CHAPTER THREE

# *DO YOUR BEST,*
# *REST (SLEEP)*
# *REPEAT*

FMS will teach you about other people, as well as yourself. I learnt to become thicker skinned, and not to worry so much about what others thought of me. I realised I had always tried so hard to protect my *reputation*, but this was underpinned by my desire to have people **like me** and think highly of me. I now operate from **character** rather than **reputation**, as reputation is what other people think of you.

However, character can bring you the same result; it just may take longer for others to come to respect your character. If they don't hang around long enough, whilst going through initial acceptance of a chronic condition, then they will never know your true character.

It is said adversity will inform you about who your true friends are and this often proved true. When I declined invitations and paced my activities (from necessity), some people moved on. Often I felt judged by others but I had to rise above this, as if these people were 'true friends' then they would offer the understanding and acceptance that was needed at that time. I was only doing what I needed to do—not what I was choosing to do. I did not intend to hurt anyone's feelings or annoy anyone by doing this—but, unfortunately I couldn't keep everyone happy, all of the time—so, due to FMS I was forced to stop trying so hard.

For all the people who 'walk out', there are some that in fact 'walk in'. And these are the people that I grabbed and held close and hope to know for a very long time. Those who walked out didn't show compassion or understanding, and I had to accept the loss. When I didn't have the capacity or strength to continue to make a big effort, then some people moved on. Sometimes, it did feel like more people were moving on than moving in, but it's about quality relationships, about depth of relationship, and not quantity.

Family is connected by blood, and as such—most (extended) family relationships are usually not affected, if you are unable to attend every activity/

gathering. There will be next time, and your 'place' will always be there—when you are able to make it. I have re discovered this recently, when I have made contact again with my extended family—after a very long time!

Family usually offer unconditional acceptance and this is useful, especially when you are not able to explain yourself or your needs, due to the unknown and lack of energy. I always encouraged Brenton and Chenoa to attend anything—even if I was unable to muster the energy.

Unless one really understands the exhaustion and fatigue that is unrelenting with FMS, then it's hard to explain. I tried to explain mine to the doctor, by using the following description 'An extreme tired feeling, but also a weighted feeling. Like there was a weight placed on the top of my head, that drags downwards through the rest of my body—until it feels like its pulling down my eyes and everything from the top down, right down to the bottoms of my feet'. To lose energy and never feel like the energy is in the body, is quite different to feeling unmotivated, uninspired or lethargic and tired—it's so much more!

I don't even bother to explain to other people anymore—but suffice to say, when people are sick with flu type symptoms, the body aches and they experience intense tiredness—it's similar to that.

The only difference is that in the case of flu or illness, this passes.

We don't often get that luxury and when and if we do—it's a matter of how long it lasts. It's never relieved by rest or sleep. AND it IS REAL!

Even conversations and social activities become increasingly difficult. Some days I couldn't even communicate or be bothered to talk. As my fatigue got worse through the day, there came the 'point of no return', where it felt like my body started to 'shut down, and talking was a part of this.

Therefore, I was not even able to talk on the phone when I felt that extreme. I couldn't be part of conversation even in small groups. It became increasingly difficult to cope, especially in highly stressful situations and/or environments—noisy, unusual lighting, cold etc. It seemed like it took every ounce of energy JUST TO BE THERE. So, then I would feel **guilty!** Then, I would worry about people feeling ignored, or being upset and not understanding my behaviour(s).

Some people understood, others did not and made me feel uncomfortable or under pressure. I realised I had to change my reaction to this, as it didn't help.

This reduced my circle of friends somewhat, as I became very selective about friendships and stuck close to those who didn't seem to have high expectations from me. At that time 'true help came from people who knew that I couldn't give anything in return'.

Getting through each day was a struggle and that's what I needed to focus my energy onto. So, I learned to ignore the phone and avoided speaking to people—not by choice BUT out of necessity! It could not be helped.

For two full years (2008, 2009) I avoided many activities and denied many social invitations. No one felt more disappointed about that, than me. I felt so many losses and felt that we were missing out on so much. Where ever possible, Chenoa and Brenton would attend—as it didn't seem fair to me that they missed out too. This was not normal behaviour for me and originally I think even Brenton was convinced I was depressed. It wasn't that at all, and he slowly came to realise that. He also slowly came to respect my decision(s) and stopped pushing me (from good intention)—to attend the things that came up. I became 'non-committal', as I was unsure how I would be feeling at that time. I stopped planning too far ahead, which was most unusual for me! These **changes** in behaviour were quite significant.

Over time, I began to realise that I was missing out on so much, and I also learned a lot about managing and pacing activities and felt more empowered. So, I began to limit and be selective BUT tried to make more effort to do things that were important. So, any social activity or event I wished to attend required some major groundwork and planning—both at work and at home. Stress around that time needed to be kept to minimum. The days before (the event/activity) I needed to ensure there were not too many physical demands on my body—for example grocery shopping etc. I needed to try to get regular rest and not take on too much. I had to be even more selective (at those times) and these extra activities had to be kept to minimum at the same time.

For example, attending the Royal Adelaide Show was an important annual family activity for us. So, the week before I would make all efforts to focus on conserving my energy. I then had to sit down with Chenoa and Brenton and 'plan' how we would do the pavilions and displays, dogs, animals etc. We had to factor in plenty of rest breaks at regular intervals. Sit down for hour stops for eating and drinking etc. We had to work around where we needed to park the car, minimise my walking distances which meant the time of day was also of consideration. But, all that even makes those 'simple' activities even more precious in my mind.

In January 2009, my immediate and close colleague was (joint) recipient of the Employee Recognition Award. As result of this, I was extremely fortunate that she and I attended a work related conference up in Surfers Paradise Qld. Now, that took some planning! All was well, but by the second day I was feeling so tired and fatigued that I struggled to eat. Nausea, light headedness and dizziness (possibly low blood pressure) was with me pretty much from the time I got up in the morning—which made it hard to get through breakfast. But, it was a great experience and very enjoyable and so that outweighed the negatives!

In April 2009, we got our little puppy! Chenoa had desperately wanted a puppy from early age and finally we took the plunge. Much research went into this puppy, and we looked into crate training etc. All the preparation and training was to make things as simple as possible in long run.

I knew I couldn't cope with a high maintenance dog, and at that age—the primary caregivers of pets are of course—the parents. We have no regrets about the puppy either—she has been a wonderful part of our family and is also an accredited DELTA therapy dog (more about this later!).

Through these difficult times we shared many memorable events and tried to make their importance very significant, as they should be—for Chenoa's sake. We had a couple of family trips to Melbourne, Chenoa's First Holy Communion, Chenoa's confirmation, Chenoa's Birthday Parties plus all the parties she attended, school holidays, time at Victor—all which required significant planning and preparation! Chenoa and I also were lucky enough to have a girls' weekend with one of her friends—where we went to Melbourne for 2 nights to see 'Mary Poppins' The Musical. We indulged in a limo, horse drawn carriage, nice dinners, fancy breakfasts and all the things that many of us do with our kids or daughters. These are the times our children remember, and why should Chenoa miss out?

In January 2008 was my 40th birthday. I had been in poor health since August/September of 2007, in the lead up to my 40th. I am not sure if it was a part of being in poor health or turning 40—or both these factors combined—but I was prompted to follow a certain path and seek people from my past, including friends from School years. The 'time' seemed right for me to do this, and became a part of enjoying my 40th celebrations and party.

Unfortunately and very sadly, this quest led me to discover that one of my very near and dear friends from my youthful years had passed away. I was devastated to learn that this dear friend had passed away from terminal illness, only a few months before I made this contact. I still feel very sad about this, and I am very disappointed that I didn't do this sooner. I felt sick for days and still feel like crying whenever I think about her. I still grieve for this dear friend and feel very sad that our opportunity to reconnect was missed. However, I also took this on board and made the decision that I had to turn things around and understand just how fragile life is, to take nothing for granted and to never live with any regrets!

Over time, since then I have reconnected with numerous extended family members as no matter what happens we should place these people and our history—of utmost importance. All these moments and memories should be truly cherished! None of us ever knows what may be around the corner, and therefore, try to make the most of every day.

As I mentioned earlier, I have also had an avid interest in community service and have always contributed and participated via Voluntary involvement. This underpins who I am—is part of my character and is important to me. There is also much to be said about what we gain from being a volunteer and by helping others less fortunate than ourselves. So, through times where 'pacing', planning, preparation and being selective were all vitally important—so, to me—was my voluntary service!

In 2010, I volunteered for 2 days for the **Special Olympics**, which were held in Adelaide. I had to be realistic about the activities I attended—determined by venue, travel distance from home, duration of the day's program, whether it was indoors or outdoors (environment), start time and finish time etc. I also had to arrange for one week of annual leave—as I knew that I wouldn't be capable of spending my 2 days off—as a volunteer at the 'Special Olympics' and then complete my usual workload.

So, my week of annual leave was approved and I planned my week accordingly. The focus of that week was the 2 (full) days I was going to spend as a much appreciated volunteer.

I was so pleased that I made this effort, as the joy and the excitement in the atmosphere and the positive attitudes were just amazing. So much spirit and determination shown—not just be the athletes but by their wonderful supporters, families etc. I got from these athletes so much more than what I gave to them, by volunteering my time!

Our puppy, when she was just over 12 months old was successful in her assessment to receive accreditation with DELTA Pet Therapy Program. I looked into this from when our puppy was very small—from my desire to continue in volunteering and also a way that I could put some time and energy into the dog, for a good cause! I began working on different training attributes I knew they would be assessing. In July 2010 we became accredited, and in September 2010 we began fortnightly visits at Hampstead Rehabilitation Centre (Residential Rehab).

Soon after we began our visiting, I sought sponsorship (financial) from a local service club. We were very grateful that The Rotary Club of Tea Tree Gully became our sponsors! We spent a year visiting at Hampstead Centre.

Then in October 2011 we began our visits at the Modbury Hospital instead, as it is in our local community and therefore a simpler task for us involving fewer issues (travel issues, time and resources).

In 2010, I had the opportunity to travel to Fiji, with 3 other girlfriends. The first half of 2010 had seen some stabilisation of blood levels, due to medications and interventions and this was a wonderful opportunity for me. Brenton had no reservations about encouraging me to go along, as he has no desire to visit Fiji as a holiday destination. Originally, I was keen to keep my time away limited to 5 days but decided without too much convincing that a full 7 days would be great medicine and would be beneficial for me in many ways. I am able to confidently report that all four of us had a wonderful time and have absolutely no regrets or negative comments as result of this trip! It was wonderful and the timing was perfect for me.

So, this is just a snapshot of some of the other aspects that helped us to get through as a Family unit and also assisted me with my ability to cope (2007-2010).

Although I have many disappointments about what we missed out on and hold frustration over losing some quality of life, I know in my heart of hearts that I have always done my best!

I may need to address at some time in the future, some frustrations and face some unresolved loss and grief issues—however, my main goal is to ensure I do my best, to try NOT to HAVE ANY REGRETS.

**Be Grateful that you don't have everything you want. If you did, you wouldn't have anything to look forward to**

**Be grateful that you don't know everything. If you did, you wouldn't have the opportunity to learn**

**Be grateful that you had difficulties because that is when you get the opportunity to grow**

**Be grateful for your limits because that is when you can find them to eliminate**

**Be grateful for your mistakes, as they will provide valuable teaching**

**Be grateful for when you are tired because that is when you may have made a difference!**

## CHAPTER FOUR

# *IT TAKES BOTH RAIN AND SUNSHINE FOR A BEAUTIFUL RAINBOW TO APPEAR!*

I have always aspired to live by upholding the '10 Indian Commandments'=

Treat the earth and all that dwell therein with respect

Remain close to the Great Spirit

Show great respect for your fellow beings

Work together for the benefit of all Mankind

Give assistance and kindness wherever needed

Do what you know to be right

Look after the wellbeing of Mind and Body

Dedicate a share of your efforts to the greater good

Be truthful and honest at all times

Take full responsibility for your actions

\*\*\*\*\*\*\*\*\*\*\*\*\*\*\*\*\*\*\*\*\*\*\*\*\*\*\*\*\*\*\*\*\*\*\*\*\*\*\*\*\*\*\*\*\*\*

**Gratitude unlocks the fullness of life.**

**It makes sense of our past, brings todays peace and creates a more positive tomorrow.**

\*\*\*\*\*\*\*\*\*\*\*\*\*\*\*\*\*\*\*\*\*\*\*\*\*\*\*\*\*\*\*\*\*\*\*\*\*\*\*\*\*\*

These 10 Indian Commandments connect to my view about 'strength of character'. These are firm foundations from which I have used to underpin my last 10 years. Although, this journey has had many twists and turns—it is only in hindsight that I look back and make sense of what I have pulled together and made. What I have made has been 'my chapter with FMS', which will now get added to my bigger **tapestry of life.** Amongst frustration, grief and sadness I have learned to be more patient. That every day does count and that we do continue to move—albeit in very small steps.

I thought many times that I wasn't making any progress, and in fact sometimes it felt like I was going backwards. I think this is common for everyone at times in their lives, not just those who are trying to live amongst health issues or ongoing chronic conditions! But, there is always good going on as well, always positive things and memories in the making. Although it often didn't feel like we were doing much, we have actually done a lot of great things.

**Be grateful for what you have and what you have achieved.**

When we look back, we have created a beautiful landscape, a part of our history. So, now I am so grateful that I can look back and reflect with some understanding and make some sense. Now I move forward. I am not defined by these experiences but they ADD to who I am and the person I will continue to grow to become.

Whilst it's easy to wallow in self-pity (and FMS and poor health ensure we don't take any easy paths), I decided that I couldn't run away from FMS, and that I couldn't move forward by avoiding it. It was real and it was going to be part of my life. I had to remain open to learning, I had to come to place of acceptance and take responsibility for my tapestry and the 'history' I wished to create and then reflect upon. All the little steps and all the time it takes to achieve these little steps eventually DO amount to something!

Suffering is a part of everyone's life, at some stage. But this part is also the part that encourages us to develop our strength of character, to find our courage, to face the difficult situation and to do our best to overcome adversity. Through suffering, we are also given the opportunity to become better people, and to grow. To be able to look back and be proud and triumphant at how far we have managed to come! ***Like the butterfly you all have the strength and hope to believe, that in time you will emerge from your cocoon . . . transformed!'***

There will be a flow of support—but sometimes we don't realise what we have at that time. Often we are disappointed as we don't receive the support from where we 'expect' and some people may let us down, or are unable to support us. However, there will be other people waiting or coming through our lives that will provide us with what we need at that time. Remember the song 'you can't always get what you want' . . . But, you usually can find 'what you need'. I knew that first I had to become my own best friend and this included nurturing my SELF.

Many things helped me to get through—to where I am today. I would say without a doubt that originally what I searched for was 'education', to inform myself and thus feel empowered about what was happening. It is this that leads to understanding, and then acceptance followed, although not at all times.

It is these tools that then ***enabled*** me, as I was able to become an active participant in managing my condition. I needed both scientific and medical intervention before making my peace via acceptance—then I could move forward.

However, the greatest key to my wellbeing was in recognising and bringing together the PHYSICAL-PSYCHOLOGICAL-SPIRITUAL elements. We are all different but YOU will find your own way—you will find your own guiding light.

I knew this condition was real and what was happening was real. However, there is only limited research and treatments available. Researchers are still developing theories and working hard in their own areas—but this will take some time. The interventions are largely defined as 'pharmalogical' and 'Non Pharmalogical' approaches, or a combination of both can be used. Overall, even now I mostly choose to use a combination of these approaches and interventions.

I knew that I couldn't afford to wait for a 'cure' or for more research to be done, more awareness, more understanding and acceptance etc. I had to start taking action. Whilst I am not a religious person, I have definitely benefitted from strengthening my spirituality. What we believe is individual and private to us but if nothing else I knew I had to find my inner strength—my own guiding light and connect with it. I think that this 'connection' to wellbeing applies to people not just with FMS, but people managing any chronic health issue, or ongoing health issues—or indeed life challenges.

I decided not to dwell on WHY this may have happened. I decided not to feel guilty about what has brought me to this point—but, rather to take back my power, focus on the future and look ahead!

With adversity I believe we develop wisdom and perseverance. We develop courage and find our own inner strength and we gain self-knowledge. We haven't necessarily (or knowingly)'chosen' this pathway, but we do have the power to choose how we react to the resulting situation. Positive thinking helps us to look at our situation with the hope that there will be some good to come out of these circumstances. Worrying and negative thinking will not assist us, and indeed may actually worsen the symptoms as well as bring down our emotional wellbeing.

***I had to learn to BE rather than DO!*** I had to slow down and work within my limits. This only came from self-knowledge and acceptance. I am still learning and developing in this regard. Undoubtedly 2007, 2008 and 2009 were my 'worst years'.

Then with 2010, came my year of stabilisation. Now, I have long term management to focus on, keeping my WELLBEING in the holistic sense, at the fore front.

When I put the Physical-psychological-spiritual **wellbeing** centre stage, it encompassed many elements.

Under the **PHYSICAL** realm, I sought information, understanding, and became involved in my health care plan. I took responsibility for restoration of my physical health. This included the reliance of medicine and medications and choosing the path towards empowerment. Reclaiming my control and following medical pathways that I felt comfortable with. It was also about trusting my own power and instincts. Learning from my GP and being involved.

I had to learn to be extremely patient, as we were only able to take small steps due to the medications and other factors involved. It took time, and I had to accept that, and focus my thoughts elsewhere instead of getting frustrated.

This also included focus on exercise. In 2007 my weight was around 68kgs. By early 2010 it reached 78kgs. It had previously (2003/2004) increased to 88kgs! Currently (Oct 2011) it's around 72 kgs and still requires a large focus within my health care and long term management. 'Exercise' is not just about increased fitness, but also about energy levels, muscle conditioning and weight management.

The physical realm also includes nutrition and this will impact on weight management. The physical realm brings together many aspects of focus. I learned to respect hormones and the influences they have on our state of mind! The physical realm obviously impacts on my overall wellbeing and is closely linked with my psychological wellbeing. Physical knowledge and physical wellness will help to keep me strong and will assist with my overall empowerment and strength. However, my physical care is only one third of the full **wellbeing** state.

Once I had an understanding of my physical health issues, I then kept up to date with information. When I felt reasonably satisfied with the fact that my physical health was moving along nicely (albeit SLOWLY), I then needed to take action in other areas that would benefit me in the longer term.

I began to focus on the **psychological realm**. To build my optimism, to become more positive, to practise mindfulness, to better manage anxiety and stress, to remain hopeful, to practice gratitude, to seek support and to focus on what my own needs were. To understand who I was and what was helpful and not helpful. I had temporarily lost sight of how important physical health really is. I had underestimated the very close connection that physical health can have on our psychological wellbeing—especially with so many elements in play. Seeking appropriate support was a vital part of getting through such difficult and challenging times. These changes or heightened awareness's also added to my depth and strength of character!

I then moved on to my **spiritual development.** But, this happened alongside the other two realms. This aspect was when my wellbeing was most improved. When all three became combined, this was when I was able to 'let go' of my job. I may always need the medications and intervention, but with all three realms working together I feel confident I will maintain my WELLBEING.

When explaining **spirituality,** this is in terms of your beliefs—your faith. Even if this is simply belief and faith in yourself! It may be about connecting to your own inner strength. It is about whatever is going to resonate with you and what is going to help you—the individual.

In my case, I hoped that by having a deep sense of personal strength I would connect to my own spiritual energy and, therefore, have the courage to live according to my own personal and highly regarded values.

For others, this may simply be the connection with 'higher self'—the inner spiritual connection deep inside. It may be considered as *the inner connection with the 'true self'*, having the higher qualities of the mind. It may be about a connection that leads the individual to peace, calm and positivity. It may be 'God'. This will be different for everyone.

The spiritual awareness that happens when we 'connect' (even if only for few minutes), is that this connection helps to keep things in perspective, to find a solution.

It may be prayer, or contemplation. It may be practising gratefulness. Spirituality may include a variety of experiences—wonder and awe, respect for nature, calmness & stillness, simplicity, tenderness, core values and individual universal truths, fulfilment and peace. Spirituality includes anything that encourages us to contemplate nature, the Divine or the Universe. Spirituality doesn't need to be complex but can be simple. It doesn't need to be religious but can be experiencing the simple things every day. I tried to engage in some activities regularly that included the beach and an appreciation of nature, meditation, reading positive books, doing my volunteering, and prayer.

Of course, faith is also part of this. **Faith** can also be considered a medicine that we can draw on, but each individual decides the dosage that best suits us. Faith has tiny wings, but can accomplish much, with our work and commitment!

When my physical and psychological aspects had been addressed, then I was able to take a huge 'leap of faith'. I had developed faith in myself. I _trusted_ that we would make sound financial decisions and if need be I would have options. But, I took this leap of faith—and resigned from the job I loved. Earlier in my journey, my job was what helped me keep perspective. It's what helped me to stay focussed and strong—to not give up. However, I began to realise that working in a job and not having a reasonable quality of life (whilst I was trying to regain my health)—was not good for me in the long term.

I knew I needed to 'surrender' (Buddhist related philosophy refers to 'patient acceptance') and trust, and I knew that the time had come for me to allow my physical health every opportunity to heal. That by allowing more time and energy for the balanced life that I wasn't used to—would in turn also boost my psychological and spiritual wellbeing.

I dearly hoped that I would be better able to participate in a more balanced lifestyle. I hoped I would be able to make time to see friends, reclaim my social life and social networks, re-establish relationships with extended family and networks, and enjoy my volunteering role(s). For our family to look ahead with the ability to plan holidays and enjoy all the future milestones, growth and learning that comes with seeing children grow up.

I realised that the working (whilst in poor health) was negatively impacting on my abilities to have any quality of life—as it took all my time and energy to get through my work (only 3 days) and minimal, daily chores at home. This meant that quality of life of the whole family was greatly diminished, which wasn't good for my long term wellbeing, nor for our family life.

I felt confident (at that point) that my psychological and spiritual developments meant that I could cope emotionally, without my job.

I had found and developed an inner strength that would help me to cope. That with these developments, then perhaps even my physical health may become slightly improved and/or restored—or in the least— better managed in long term.

I did feel the judgements of others and hear people say how 'lucky' I was that I was able to make such a decision. I agree I have much to be grateful for, however, it's not necessarily the decision I wanted to make. But, I also knew it was the right decision for us to make as a family.

There would be different positives in our lives if I was able to continue to contribute to our household income, but we have never generated a highly materialistic lifestyle and we felt confident that we would have the capacity to cope for a while. One cannot put a price on wellbeing and the solid foundation and happiness of family life. I became good at ignoring what other people perceived of our situation, without being appropriately informed or qualified.

My health and wellbeing impacts directly on our home and family life—and right now that's my priority and what is most important to us. I am now better informed and know to 'pace' activities and this will add to and ensure my 'participation' and Quality of Life. These will have a flow on effect and hopefully further enhance our family life and family happiness. Our household finances will determine and directly influence this current situation, but I am minimalist by nature. I loathe shopping and shopping centres and love being in nature! I love the 'simple things'. Lucky for me, the best things in life are free! Much can be done on a tighter and restricted budget, if the energy can be mustered up!

I felt that I had made a huge shift in my thinking. Perhaps I had reached some (patient) acceptance of the long term physical impacts resulting from FMS.

I now had the inclination to restore some quality of life. Those people who are important in our lives and valuable to our family know and understand the true meaning and depth underpinning our decisions over the last 12 months.

So, I confidently now inform you all that as well as strengthening the PHYSICAL-PSYCHOLOGICAL-SPIRITUAL connection, I also understand it! I also know that these elements—all together—add up to individual WELLBEING.

As well as making this connection and learning a lot along the way, I am also proud to inform you that I have developed my *__'strength of character__'* through this journey.

*Strength of character* may be described as having the inner strength (spirit) to do what you know is right, even when it's difficult to do so. It's different to reputation, which is what others think of you. Instead of focussing on what others think, strength of character means we focus on **who we really are!**

It's about accepting responsibility for who and what you become. It's about adversity and challenge. It's about 'finding' your own courage to face these situations.

**Strength of character** is also your mark on the world. This mark on the world IS your impact. It's doing the right thing, even if you don't feel like it (illness), even if it's inconvenient, even if no one is looking, even if it costs friendships, and even if no one understands . . . . Any of this sound familiar ??

## Chapter Five

# Looking Ahead— The Four Of Us

Throughout my life, I have always been very independent (mostly from necessity), and in many ways Brenton has been much the same. We had each managed on our own, in our own worlds until we met up, just over 14 years ago! Then, we had our daughter and together we have managed to get through without much support or intervention from others. This was predominantly by our own choice, whether this was the 'right' choice is now irrelevant as we have managed to get to this point.

Then, we had our family of three (with Chenoa) and then this went up by another one—with our family pet. We have always tried to live within our means, and have refrained from competing with others or 'wanting' what we couldn't afford. We have made the most of family life and Brenton and I truly count our blessings, that we have our 'tight family unit'.

Brenton has always accepted me for who I am. He has always gone with 'the flow' with my choice of profession, employment, volunteer work etc. When I became unwell—he allowed me the space to deal with it in my own way. I'm sure it was hard for him to watch me go through these difficulties. He would have liked to 'fix it', or have some 'miracle pill' to make it all go away—so we could return to our life. In time, I guess he realised (as well as me) that we had a new reality to manage within.

When Brenton and I first met I was very proactive, and was (still am in spirit) a workaholic by nature. Always gave 100% commitment, never gave up and always worked at something until I achieved the desired result. It has helped our relationship that he has seen my capabilities 'pre FMS'. He has never doubted what is going on for me, although I know he has often felt helpless. But, he just kept going—doing what he needed to do to fulfil his responsibilities—as a partner and a father.

Because he knew me 'pre FMS' he knew that by nature I 'wasn't a lazy person'—as I wouldn't have survived in my life. I had always been a 'do—er', getting things done. Never asked for help or expected help from others. So, he KNEW deep down, that this poor state of health wasn't in my mind and it was very real. It was indeed real for all of us.

Then, he watched me go through some difficult times—often not knowing what to do or how to help. He did what he could to relieve pressure from me and to ensure Chenoa's childhood was filled with the stability and parenting that she deserved. At times, he needed to 'make up' for my share as well. Indeed, to make up for the parent that at times, I wasn't able to be for her.

Through those times, he simply accepted without question all the therapies; alternatives etc I sought help from. He remained open minded and encouraging. He didn't necessarily 'believe' in the positive effects of all these resources, but he would listen to what I disclosed and allow me to get on with it all—in my own way. Although, he also knew me well enough to know that I was of strong, determined character and wouldn't step away from things just because he didn't agree.

But his open and accepting attitude did make things easier and simpler at that time. He encouraged me to look at crystals, to do scrapbooking, to read the books etc. I didn't ever feel I needed to justify any of it to him but by the same token—he had trust in me that I 'would always do what was right'.

I know that at times I would have frustrated him no end. Sometimes he did frustrate me. Sometimes I felt (at that time) that it may have been helpful if he had looked into the condition and the affects etc. We have certainly had our own relationship tension, and difficulties to work through. But, overall he has coped in his own way and I have also had to allow that. He showed me great respect, and I needed to do the same. Through all of this the ups and downs—he, like me—has always done his best—I have never doubted that.

Without these challenges, our family life may have unfolded differently. However, between us and our similar values we have built a solid family foundation. Together, through these experiences we have been there for each other. We have offered each other unconditional love, good solid stability, sound support and the greatest acceptance!

We have created, over time and through challenges—our own family history—for the three (four) of us. We have a responsibility and commitment to continue on, in the future and continue to build our future history.

Our wonderful daughter has also come through difficult times in a positive way—due to our determined efforts and unrelenting love and commitment to her. Since I left my job, the extra time and (sometimes minimal and always fluctuating) energy I have had, has assisted with her schooling and lifted some of her results. She continues to 'do her best' and this is all we expect, and time and time again we have discussed this with her. As her parents we have demonstrated it to her over her early years. She has a passion for horses, dogs and animals and has an ever growing love of horse riding. She dreams of one day having her own horse and has dreams and plans of her own future. She is making her own way and we support her to follow her passions and interests and encourage her to find her own 'guiding light within'.

She has a great love of reading, (as I always have had) and we also nurture and encourage this. In fact, as I write this—she is also writing her own fictional story! She also sets herself a desired goal and will work diligently to achieve her outcome. She is very creative and has a vivid imagination, which she engages with whenever the opportunity presents! She is very balanced and happy within herself and this has been from the input of both of us—in different ways. We still have years ahead of parenting and guiding this wonderful child and I speak for both of us, when I say we intend to enjoy the experience while it lasts! Chenoa knows her own mind and can stand up for her beliefs and rights. Chenoa and I have often gone 'head to head'. But, I believe this is healthy, as it encourages her to explore her ideas and at times we agree to disagree.

On the flip side, she is also a warm, caring, compassionate person who is wise beyond her years. Yes, the last five years have played a big part in her life and will influence her future BUT we have done OK. I know there have been times of uncertainty and this may have caused her concern. At times she lacked the capacity to understand what has been happening. But, I have always tried to communicate with her to ensure she is OK and Brenton has provided the 'extra' care when needed.

Her care has never been jeopardised, and her state of mind and wellbeing has always been of utmost importance of us both.

I have always made my best efforts to be there for important activities, made sure she has had opportunities to do what she loves—albeit sometimes not quite in the way I would have hoped or anticipated/expected. Usually, Brenton and I have both proudly been able to witness the milestones and events and activities of great importance to her. We are grateful for those privileges!

One Saturday (late 2011), Chenoa and I attended a local church craft fair/market—at her request. She was very happy to receive two items, without spending a cent! She was given two separate 'gifts' by two different people—for just being her self. What a great boost to her self-esteem and confidence. What a reward to be proud of. How special is that! I am truly grateful to those women for also being so generous and kind to our beautiful child.

When I think of myself, I think about what lead me to start writing and hope that this makes publication (printing), and in turn helps a few people out there in this huge world.

I recently looked at the book I have been diligently recording results, outcomes of doctors' visits etc. Of significance is that a soft cover book (exercise type book) was given to me in late 2008, by a friend in the workplace—who knew of my difficulties. On the back cover, the following sentence is scrawled

**'IT IS HERE WHERE SHE MUST BEGIN TO TELL HER STORY'** . . .

I had never before noticed this! And the day after I decide to write 'our story', I notice such an important message . . . seems like it was mapped out before I knew of it?

Late in 2011 I was asked to consider a job share position, within community services once again. I had much apprehension, although the position was only for a possible 15 hours/week from early 2012.

The opportunity prompted me to again think of our future (paid employment) and our household financial position. Brenton always remains happy with whatever decision we make. Chenoa, on the other hand makes it quite clear that she hopes I can be around (emotionally and physically) as I have been for the last 12 months—without being totally exhausted by school pick up time. I have concerns over my quality of life—which stem from concerns about my reduced capacity and reduced ability to cope. I am not quite 'there' yet!

I am of the thinking that, along with the hours I assist with supporting our business and household, the maximum I could manage would be 10 hours per week in another job role. I feel that if I exceed that limit, I will again jeopardise my long term wellbeing, due to not managing my condition in the best way for me. I need to weigh up the benefits, the finances and the long term management of my physical health, as well as the long term wellbeing of our family life. The latter two are the most important—to all of us—even the dog!

We are very excited that finally we will venture outside of this state of South Australia. Chenoa hasn't been on many family 'holidays' for the last 6 or 7 years.

We recently travelled to Sydney late 2011, to celebrate Brentons 50th Birthday! Later this year we intend to take Chenoa to the snow—which the three of us have never had the opportunity to do. We are even planning a BIG road trip, up along NSW coastline and up to Queensland—where we will spend 5 days on the Gold Coast (Surfers Paradise). This will take a lot of planning—financially, emotionally, practically and physically—but we are pretty sure we will do it—before Chenoa becomes a teenager!

My walks get longer and my first 8 km walk was achieved a few months ago—at Victor Harbor. I managed a walk that I have not been able to do for around 6 years! I was very proud of myself.

I have made the same walk—one way approx. 12 months ago but not both ways (4kms each way). I did it and it felt good—but I experienced a false sense of success.

I also experienced a flare up and dramatic step backwards (relapse)—around 4 days afterwards (which lasted around 5 days). So, maybe I am not quite able to make that yet—maybe a little too much for me. I may be able to achieve this in another few months or maybe never. Maybe it will be a case of weighing up the outcome versus reward. Maybe I will enjoy the sense of achievement whilst understanding that I will 'pay' for it later on. Surely it won't hurt every now and again?

## CHAPTER SIX

# DESTINATION UNKNOWN!

## WHERE TO FROM HERE?

None of us really knows where we may be heading next. But, I do know a couple of very important things . . . .

Firstly, True spiritual growth will happen when an acceptance of suffering is realised. If we surrender to the suffering we allow true experiences in life to be fulfilling. I am not saying that FMS is a fun time to be enjoyed. But, pain and suffering are a part of life and many people struggle with these aspects of life. I was (am) no different. Instead of enduring my suffering and becoming miserable, over time I learned to take these challenges as an opportunity to grow and to learn about patience, balance and self-acceptance. It has become an opportunity for HEALING.

Secondly, I believe in divine timing, synchronicity or providence and many elements fell into place, at the right time. It is a *process* and I couldn't skip ahead—no matter how much I wanted to. I maintained my trust along with the hope that things would get better. I wasn't in the right place or right frame of mind earlier on—to deal with everything the way I feel I can now. I also wanted to follow this path, as I knew I had to find another way. Growth doesn't work if the student isn't ready—you cannot be told when and how to develop these things—you have to make your own way. When the student is ready—the teacher appears! That is what I believed and my faith (as another medicine) got me through in regular doses, and assisted me to take necessary actions. I now feel more confident than I have for a long time!

Thirdly, we will face whatever comes our way—together as a strengthened Family Unit.

***Family*** *is the first social unit for developing the qualities of the heart. A true **family** grows and moves through life together, inseparable in the heart. Whether a biological family or an extended family of people attracted to each other based on heart resonance and mutual support, the word "**family**" implies warmth, a place where the core feelings of the heart are nurtured. **Family** values represent the core values and guidelines that parents and family members hold in high regard for the well-being of the **family**. Sincere **family** feelings are* *core heart feelings. They are the basis for true **family** values. While we have differences, we remain "**family**" by virtue of our heart connection. **Family** provides necessary security and support, and acts as a buffer against external problems. A **family** made up of secure people generates a magnetic power that can get things done. They are the hope for real security in a stressful world.*

Finally, I intend to treasure and hold close to me the valuable gifts of learning that I have received through this time. None of it has been for nothing.

*Which aspect do I think has helped the most—the Physical, the psychological or the spiritual?*

Now, that's hard to say. But I will say this . . .

Within the physical element, I need to maintain good nutrition and exercise. As well as learn my limits regarding physical demands. It's really no different to a person that has recovered from a shoulder injury— if they exceed a certain level—then the end result is pain and flare up. They learn they have done too much. A person with diabetes learns to maintain a diet and learns their boundaries of what is 'likely' to have a negative affect or consequence. These people also learn how to cope. They learn how to manage in the long term. Our physical health is no different when we are trying to manage FMS, or other conditions which relate to energy stores and production. We will have a pain threshold and activity limits that we need to remain within—or pay the consequences. We need to take adequate steps with sleep maintenance, medication, diet, nutrition and exercise. Maybe for a while we just need to dedicate more focus to these areas and accept any limitations. These important areas need to become our 'work' and we need to respect and love ourselves enough to dedicate time, effort and energy to these areas—and possibly even make some lifestyle changes!

In regards to our psychological health, I can speak most positively about the difference made by changing to a more optimistic way of thinking and viewing the world. To develop strength of character will lead us into new worlds.

I believe that our biggest successes will come from within the networks that we are known (for example 'our' community). Character and personal integrity adds to reputation. People are always watching. We develop networks and relationships around us, and this in itself will provide more opportunities for us—word of mouth is the best way to promote and sell yourself and your strengths, and over time with consistent and persistent effort—the rewards will come. It will be the optimistic thinking and positive thoughts that will find them or make the opportunities good things . . . It's all about our perspective and patience!

Spiritually, I have always believed in timing, in divine guidance, Providence. Although I am still not sure exactly what that means for me—I know there is something bigger than us. The Universe (God) works in amazing ways.

Once we raise our (spiritual) energy and shift our thinking, then so many doors will open and opportunities will come our way. One thing will lead to the next thing and we will be on our way. I learned to trust this process.

Once we start to give, by way of volunteering or helping others, and being grateful, if the motivation is genuine and from the heart, then stick with it. Eventually it will come back to you. Today is another day we have been given—Enjoy it, as life is a gift!

But, I can assure you that it's not enough to just have faith or optimism or science or medicine to 'rely on'. That won't bring us the help we need to improve our 'wellbeing'. The doorbell wont ring with everything delivered. The opportunities and the stepping stones are there, BUT we have to find them. We have to search and undertake the action that will start this flow of events. If we don't take the action, then we will stay where we are. We may take every medication known to man and still may not feel great.

We still need to do the hardest work—it's not just learning or 'knowing' it's also about action and 'doing'. Sounds hard? Well, it is but don't get disheartened, as it does get easier. I know how hard it can be . . . How frustrating, annoying, painful, upsetting, lonely, isolating and so on and so forth—as many experiences can be. But, never give up!

Find the strength and courage to get up again the next day, and take the next steps, one foot in front of the other, one at a time, one day at a time. Eventually you will look back and see how far you have come— like I have. Yes, I feel like I have lost many things. But, also many wonderful things have been gained. It's not necessarily any worse—it's just different. Just try to do your best, with what you have at each step of the way. Be kind to yourself and get to know yourself.

Therefore, it is my opinion that neither area is more important, helpful or useful.

BUT, they are all as equally important for my WELLBEING—with my individual action and input!

I wish you well and above all,

*I hope you always find your strength, courage, hope and faith!*

## **<u>To BELIEVE . . .</u>**

# Afterword

Around 7/8 months have now passed since completing the original writing and first draft. Although I started writing and it all came together quickly (thanks to my journaling over many years!)—I still didn't know if it would end up becoming published. Once finished I looked into publishing options, packages etc. From there I asked 2 people to read the initial draft. Due to great encouragement and feedback, I then investigated possible sources of financial support and sponsorship to try to 'make it happen'. My facebook page ('Fibromyalgia Wellbeing') was created, and continues to grow way beyond my expectations—thus, bringing us to where we are today. It has been clearly demonstrated that there is a great need for support and better understanding in regards to Fibromyalgia.

Since completing the initial draft I continue to learn and make positive changes each day. However, I still encounter frequent setbacks and acute episodes of illness and flare up(s). For example, the first 3 months of this year (2012) I experienced 3 significant sinus infections—one per month. So, out of 12 weeks, I was at various levels of being unwell for six weeks—half of that time! I still struggle with these episodes and, as yet—don't have all the answers.

In January this year (2012) we purchased a slow cooker and a low cost juice extractor. I have religiously used both of these and learned many things along the way. I have always had an interest in juicing but now have come to view diet, nutrition and all the related processes of very high importance in my treatment plan. I now use food as a medicine and consider nutritional medicine will lead to a good result. I am now an avid 'fan' of fresh veggie juicing and loads of veggies and high intake of nutritional foods. Certainly on the flip side, we also need to know about our intolerances and what foods we should avoid when we have chronic health problems. I continue with (almost) daily exercise. And I am pleased to report that my appropriate medical care, support and intervention have also resulted in my medication and blood results becoming more stable and consistent.

All of this together equates to a lot of time and effort (action)—exercise regime equates to 15-25 minutes almost every day (followed by shower); juicing prep and clean up equates to approx. half an hour—with rest breaks in between, then there is meal/diet considerations. Some days it comes easier than others, some days I don't feel like doing these 'routines' (and the work) but do it anyway. Some days I am simply not well enough to do these things on top of take adequate care of the minimal things at home and get the rest that my body needs. So, on those days I rest when possible, and try to be gentle on myself. I hope that it will pass, and that tomorrow I will be able to pick it all up again. I now accept it better when the latter happens, as I continue to do my best WHEN I can. Sometimes life is too busy and these 'routines' further add to my stress levels, so I reduce my outputs and outcomes accordingly.

However, the positive outcome makes it all worth the effort! I AM WORTH THE EFFORT . . . I still have a long way to go, but each time I come back from a bad spell, I find I am bouncing back quicker and each time—I come back a little stronger, feeling a little better and less exhausted and fatigued. I know I am again moving forwards in this regard. So now, if I can just make the good bits last longer than the bad I will be most happy! These new routines and behaviours are becoming more ingrained and hopefully will become less like work and more like 'habits'. But, for now—they are PRIORITIES.

I am also happy to announce that a couple of months ago I was offered another part time position, back in the area of CARER SUPPORT. The position was offered to me, with the flexibility and nurturing that is needed for at least the near future, whilst I continue to 'work' on my health. The position is also minimal hours and happily I accepted. It is also finances from this paid job role that will enable this book to become published! However, when I was considering the pro's and con's I had much to consider. I had to work out if I could maintain a good balance and continue to support my wellbeing and wellness.

Part of this was to employ a cleaner, on a fortnightly basis. We don't have a large home but she is able to do in 3 hours what I had to do over two days due to physical limitations! So, having this cleaning support is a positive change and one that has been very welcome and reflective about valuing my physical needs. I am able to pay the cost, from the income that I will now earn, and further simplify my workload in physical sense. I now demonstrate that I value myself and I consider that I deserve this opportunity to focus on my health needs and that I am worthy of this help.

As well as these developments, I have also learned to speak my truth and communicate my needs better. I have found my voice when it comes to boundaries and preserving my health. I've come to realise this is NOT selfish behaviour, but indeed responsible behaviour. Although I don't consider I was a 'bad' person, I now learn to slowly let go of old patterns and behaviours that may not be in my best interests.

I now embrace a new 'reality' and let go of the outdated. I have slowly overcome (and let go of) many fears and still continue to address contributing stress. Louise Hay would be proud! I still face fears and stress everyday—this is inevitable. Fear and stress can be motivating and can help keep us safe. It's whether the fear and stress is productive, appropriate and constructively managed that is the question. For example I am fearful of again putting on weight and facing additional challenges/issues. I sometimes feel stressed by the extra work involved in taking care of my diet and nutrition needs at the moment. However, these factors also motivate me to do my best to stay focussed and on track, to ensure these elements remain for now of utmost priority. The stress is alleviated as I believe that if I remain on track my overall health and wellbeing will positively benefit. If I put on weight and again face weight management issues, I will know that I haven't been honouring my body and supporting its needs. This is just something I have to do—at least until my body is more restored and replenished. These fears and stresses (and stressors) will continue to change as my life changes and I continue to grow.

I have accepted that I am a beautiful soul. I AM ME. On so many levels, I haven't changed. But, some of the outer behaviours, thought patterns and responses needed adaptation for me to have the best chance of living with optimal wellbeing. This is NOT selfish. These changes were necessary to make way for the improved lifestyle I currently need. I have had to let go of what no longer served my best interest. However, I AM STILL ME! I still need to practise hard and learn in these areas too.

This illness and accompanying health issues have forced me to find a new way. As it turns out—I believe it's actually a better way! Not just for me, but also for those around me—so how can all this imply *selfishness*?

This all doesn't mean that I wasn't doing 'well' before—but simply means I was doing the best that I could at that time—with the resources and knowledge I had. Now, I know different. I live in the present and through being confronted with health related issues, I have been prompted to learn a different way. A necessary way to try; if I hope to cope.

In Middle of March (once publishing was sorted and a certainty) I bumped into someone at the local shops that I hadn't had contact with for around 7 years. We actually originally met and became friends through 'Weight Watchers'—pre FMS diagnosis. We chatted briefly for a few minutes and I disclosed that I had been addressing some health problems and then shared with her the book project and self-publishing. She was extremely flattering and encouraging and gave me the biggest compliment that I will treasure.

I hadn't thought too much about the bigger picture of the last few years—in terms of the perspective of what I had achieved. Initially her response was 'Good for You and good on you for wanting to reach out and help others'. But then she added 'And Congratulations—for choosing to make lemonade when life gave you lemons!'

I guess to some readers and 'outsiders' it may come across this way and I proudly reflect on the hard work I have put in for myself and then look at and embrace the bigger picture.

To the people closest to me—I'm pretty sure it seems like I spend my time making their life more difficult, and at times become a pain in the backside for them. Due to their first-hand experience with—my strict limitations, endless discussions about boundaries that need to be set (at least for now), and my reduced/adjusted capabilities etc etc etc. They experience the frustration; the ups and downs, and have had to find their own ways to cope as well. Yes, I am thinking 'pain in the backside' is quite an accurate description of me for them to have!

However, for me—this is an opportunity to learn, to grow and to change. To do what needs to be done. The bottom line is that I am working towards my ultimate goal, which is to HEAL—from the INSIDE (to the outside)!

I don't really know yet if I consider the symptoms and this condition can come to a point of 'recovery' in an individual. But, I guess it depends on how 'recovery' is defined and interpreted. Many symptoms may have manifested over many decades. Maybe this damage can't be UNDONE.

But, we can aim for a better today and a much improved tomorrow. The body is truly an amazing thing! Never underestimate what it's capable of. I also know that the physical symptoms and issues presenting are REAL, no matter how they got there. However, they are also greatly influenced by our psychological and spiritual wellbeing.

I CAN achieve a good state of 'fibromyalgia wellbeing'. Some issues may always exist for me, in relation to my health—BUT, hopefully they will move to the background instead of the foreground. It may be only baby steps, it may take a long time—this will depend on many factors along the way.

With the right medical care and intervention, good nutrition, exercise, knowledge, appropriate and adequate emotional support, societal awareness and validation, behaviour, commitment, willingness to learn, an open ness to try different approaches, sound stress management, lifestyle changes . . .

BUT MOST OF ALL

**POSITIVE ATTITUDE AND SELF LOVE—**

Amazing things may truly become possible!

AND lots of lemonade may be made!!

(I may even learn to like lemonade!!!!).

\*\*\*\*\*\*\*\*\*\*\*\*\*\*\*\*\*\*\*\*\*\*\*\*\*\*\*\*\*\*\*\*\*\*\*\*\*\*\*\*\*\*\*\*\*\*\*\*\*\*\*\*\*

THIS IS NOT THE BEGINNING OF THE END,

IT'S THE RETURN TO YOURSELF.

THE RETURN TO INNOCENCE!

*Feel it—EMOTION* . . . .

*'Don't be afraid to be weak . . . don't be too proud to be strong . . . Just look into your heart my friend . . .*

*THAT WILL BE THE RETURN TO YOURSELF, THE RETURN TO INNOCENCE . . .*

*If you must . . . then start to cry . . . . just believe in destiny*

*Don't care what people say ...just follow your own way ...*

*dont give up and use the chance*

*TO RETURN TO INNOCENCE'.*

(WORDS FROM ENIGMA song 'Return to Innocence')

# APPENDIX ONE

## FROM FATIGUED TO FANTASTIC!
## YOU CAN EFFECTIVELY TREAT CFS, FATIGUE, FIBROMYALGIA, ME AND MUSCLE PAIN
### BY JACOB TEITELBAUM, MD

The "perfect storm" for fibromyalgia, chronic fatigue syndrome, and fatigue in general is preparing to hit.

A combination of poor nutrition, decreasing sleep, increasing stress and environmental toxins has created a human energy crisis of unprecedented proportions. Over the past 10 years the incidence of chronic fatigue syndrome (CFS) and fibromyalgia (FMS) has exploded by 400-1,000 percent, as documented in five separate studies. The numbers for those with CFS in the U.S., previously estimated at 500,000, are now being re-tallied at closer to 1-2.5 million. Previous estimates placed the number of Americans with fibromyalgia at 6 million, whereas more recent studies worldwide suggest this has likely gone up in the last decade to 12-24 million! Meanwhile, one quarter of Americans suffer with chronic pain, and most are fatigued.

## RESEARCH SHOWS CFS AND FIBROMYALGIA IS REAL AND TREATABLE

After decades of hard work by hundreds of researchers in the field, we have progressed to the point where effective treatment is now available for these illnesses! I led one such research study that was published as the lead article in an issue of the Journal of Chronic Fatigue Syndrome. Titled "Effective Treatment of Chronic Fatigue Syndrome and Fibromyalgia — the Results of a Randomized, Double-Blind, Placebo-Controlled Study," our study showed that 91 percent of patients improved with treatment (full text of study available at www.EndFatigue.com).

On average, patients in our study showed a 90% improvement in quality of life after only two years of treatment. Pain decreased by an average of over 50 percent (interestingly, many of the same principles for treating fibromyalgia also apply to myofascial pain syndrome, or MPS). Many patients no longer even qualified for the diagnosis of CFS or fibromyalgia after treatment!

That the vast majority of patients improved significantly in the active group while there was minimal improvement in the placebo group proved two very important things. The first is that these are very treatable diseases. The second is that anyone who now says that these illnesses are not real or are all in your head are clearly both wrong and unscientific.

A new day is dawning in how CFS, fibromyalgia and MPS will be treated. In support of our work, an editorial in the April, 2002 journal of a major multidisciplinary medical society for pain management in the U.S. noted that "the comprehensive and aggressive metabolic approach to treatment detailed in the Teitelbaum study are all highly successful approaches and make fibromyalgia a very treatment responsive disorder. The study by Dr. Teitelbaum et al. and years of clinical experience make this approach an excellent and powerfully effective part of the standard of practice for treatment of people who suffer from fibromyalgia and myofascial pain syndrome."

It is important to recognize that these syndromes can be caused and aggravated by a large number of different triggers. When all these different contributing factors are looked for, and treated effectively, patients improve significantly and often get well!

## What is Causing These Illnesses?

CFS, fibromyalgia and MPS are not a single illness. Our study has shown that they are a mix of many different processes that can be triggered by many causes. Some patients had their illness caused by any of a number of infections. In this situation, many people can identify the time that their illness began almost to the day. This is also the case in those patients who had an injury (sometimes very mild) that was enough to disrupt their sleep and trigger this process. In others the illness had a more gradual onset. This may have been associated with hormonal deficiencies (e.g., low thyroid, estrogen, testosterone, cortisone, etc.) despite normal blood tests. In others, it may be associated with chronic stress, antibiotic use with secondary yeast overgrowth, and/or nutritional deficiencies. Indeed, we have found well over 100 common causes of, and factors that contribute to, these syndromes.

What these processes have in common is that most of them can suppress a major control center in your brain called the hypothalamus. This center controls sleep, your hormonal system, temperature, and blood flow/pressure. When you don't sleep deeply, your immune system also stops working properly and you'll be in pain. When we realized this, the myriad symptoms seen in CFS and fibromyalgia suddenly made sense. It also gave us a way to effectively treat you!

## THE "S.H.I.N.E. PROTOCOL"—FIVE PROBLEM AREAS THAT NEED TO BE TREATED

A half-century of work by Dr. Janet Travell, the White House physician for Presidents Kennedy and Johnson and author of the Trigger Point Manual showed that the same problems caused by hypothalamic suppression result in muscles getting stuck in the shortened position. Chronic muscle shortening then causes myofascial and fibromyalgia pain, with chronic pain then being amplified in the brain (called Central Sensitization). As she laid the groundwork for effective treatments of these processes, our research team dedicated our published study to her memory. The following are the five key areas represented by the acronym S.H.I.N.E. that need to be treated for CFS, fibromyalgia and muscle pain to resolve:

1. **S**leep. Most patients with these illnesses find that they are unable to get 7-8 hours of deep sleep a night without taking medications. In part, this occurs because hypothalamic function is critical to deep sleep. Unfortunately, many of

the most common sleep medications actually aggravate the sleep problems by decreasing the amount of time spent in deep sleep. For patients to get well, it is critical that they take enough of the correct sleep medications to get 8 to 9 hours sleep at night! These medications include Ambien, Desyrel, Neurontin, Klonopin, and, if you don't have Restless Leg Syndrome, Flexeril and/or Elavil. In addition, natural remedies can help sleep. Effective natural remedies include those that contain theanine, Jamaican Dogwood, wild lettuce, valerian, passionflower, hops, magnesium and melatonin. In the first six months of treatment, it is not uncommon for patients to need to take as many as eight different products simultaneously to get 8 hours of sleep at night. After 6-18 months of feeling well, most people can come off of the sleep (and other) medications. (I'm starting to believe that to offer a margin of safety during periods of stress, it may be wise to stay on 1/2 to 1 tablet of a sleep medication for the rest of your life).

2.  **H**ormonal deficiencies. The hypothalamus is the main control center for most of the glands in your body. Most of the normal ranges for our blood tests were not developed in the context of hypothalamic suppression or these syndromes. Because of this (and for a number of other reasons) it is usually necessary, albeit controversial, to treat with thyroid, adrenal (very low dose cortef DHEA), and ovarian and testicular hormones — despite what normal blood tests suggest! (These hormones have been found to be reasonably safe when used in low doses.)

3.  **I**nfections. Many studies have shown immune system dysfunction in CFS and fibromyalgia. Although there are many causes of this, I suspect that poor sleep is a major contributor. The immune dysfunction can result in many unusual infections. These include viral infections (e.g., XMRV, HHV-6, CMV, and EBV, etc.), parasites and other bowel infections, infections sensitive to long-term treatment

with the antibiotics Cipro and Doxycycline (e.g., mycoplasma, chlamydia, Lyme's, etc.) and fungal infections. Avoiding sweets (though stevia is OK) and taking probiotics can be very helpful. We often also add prescription antifungals as well.

4.  **N**utritional supplementation. Because the western diet has been highly processed, nutritional deficiencies are a common problem. In addition, bowel infections can cause poor absorption, and the illness itself can cause increased nutritional needs. The most important nutrients include vitamins B and B12 (especially important), antioxidants such as vitamin C and E, minerals (especially magnesium, zinc, and selenium) and amino acids (proteins).

In addition, a newly discovered nutrient called ribose is emerging as possibly the most exciting discovery in energy research of the decade. Two studies using ribose in 300 CFS/FMS patients at 53 medical centers showed that it increased energy in patients an average of 60% after only 3 weeks!

5. <u>E</u>xercise as tolerated. In the beginning, walk as much as you can so that you feel "good tired" afterwards — meaning comfortably recovering the day of exercise and better still the next day. Because you do not yet have the energy to condition, do not push beyond what is comfortable. Otherwise, you're likely to crash. After 10 weeks on the program, your energy production will increase and you'll be able to condition by increasing your walking by one minute a day as able. When you progress to one hour a day, you can increase the intensity of your exercise.

## GETTING THE HELP YOU NEED

I would begin with the free Symptom Analysis program at Dr. Teitelbaum's website www.Endfatigue. com which will analyze your symptoms (and also pertinent lab tests if available) to:

1 - Determine the causes of your CFS/FMS/ME and

2 - Tailor a treatment protocol to your specific case. This will often give you all the information needed to get well.

Dr. Teitelbaum is also available for consultations in person in Hawaii or by phone worldwide. Holistic physicians worldwide can also help. If in the US, Fibromyalgia and Fatigue Center physicians nationwide are familiar with the SHINE protocol (www.fibroandfatigue.com)

Effective treatment is now available. It's time for people to get well!

Love and Blessings

Jacob E Teitelbaum, MD

(SUBMITTED BY Jacob E Teitelbaum, MD and used with permission* Feb 2012)

Jacob Teitelbaum, MD, is medical director of the national Fibromyalgia and Fatigue Centers and Chronicity, author of the popular free iPhone application "Cures A-Z," and author of the best-selling CFS/FMS guidebook From Fatigued to Fantastic! (Avery/Penguin Group) and Pain Free 1-2-

3-A Proven Program for Eliminating Chronic Pain Now (McGraw-Hill), Beat Sugar Addiction NOW! (Fairwinds Press, 2010, Real Cause, Real Cure (Rodale Press, July 15, 2011. Available at www.realcauserealcure. com), and the Beat Sugar Addiction NOW! Cookbook (Fairwinds, Jan 2012). Dr. Teitelbaum does frequent media appearances including Good Morning America, CNN, Fox News Channel, the Dr Oz Show and Oprah & Friends. He lives in Kona, Hawaii. Web site: www.EndFatigue.com

# Appendix Two

## Positive And Useful Quotes To Ponder

The unexamined life is not worth living (Socrates).

Wellbeing is the ultimate aim of life.

Success comes from knowing you have done your best.

There is nothing either good or bad but thinking makes it so (Shakespeare).

In understanding WELLBEING we acknowledge that every thought, word and behaviour impact on our health and wellbeing. Thus, we may be affected physically, psychologically and spiritually.

Life is what happens to you while you're busy making other plans (John Lennon).

Time is your life . . . how you spend it is how you spend your life.

For every minute you remain angry, you give up sixty seconds of peace of mind (Ralph Waldo Emerson).

Faith makes everything possible.

When hard times are upon you, you can let it make you bitter, or use it to make you better.

Keep your mind on the things you want; and off the things you don't want.

If you do your best the worst will not happen.

It's easy to be pleasant when life flows like a song; but the person worthwhile is the person who will smile when things go wrong.

The greatest of all power is the power of faith.

Never look at what you have lost—look at what you have left.

The game of life is not so much in holding a good hand—as playing a poor hand well.

If you cannot do great things, you can at least do small things in a great way.

Pain and suffering is inevitable, but misery is optional.

God grant me the serenity to accept the things
I cannot change, courage to change the things I
can—and wisdom to know the difference.

Faith is taking that first step, even when you can't
see the staircase.

When life is sweet, say thank you and celebrate.
And when life is bitter, say thank you and grow.

Choose your thoughts carefully. Keep what brings
you peace, release what brings you suffering. And
know that happiness is just a thought away!

A good plan of today is better than a great plan of
tomorrow. Look backward with satisfaction & look
forward with confidence.

The best thing to give to your enemy is forgiveness;
to an opponent, tolerance; to a friend, your
heart; to your child, a good example; to a father,
deference; to your mother, conduct that will make
her proud of you; to yourself, respect; to all men,
charity. (Francis Maitland Balfour)

As you slide down the bannisters of life, may the
splinters never point in the wrong direction
(An Irish Blessing)

Thanks to those who disliked me, you taught me
to rise above drama. To those who loved me, you

made my heart grow fonder. To those who cared, you showed me you're true. To those who entered my life, you showed me there are still good people out there. To those who left, you showed me that nothing lasts forever. To those who stayed, you showed me the meaning of a bond. To those who listened, you made me feel I was worth listening to.

By associating with wise people you will become wise yourself.

Your sacred space is where you can find yourself again and again.

This is my wish for you: Comfort on difficult days, smiles when sadness intrudes, rainbows to follow the clouds, laughter to kiss your lips, sunsets to warm your heart, hugs when spirits sag, beauty for your eyes to see, friendships to brighten your being, faith so that you can believe, confidence for when you doubt, courage to know yourself, patience to accept the truth, Love to complete your life.

### YOU ARE—

You are strong . . . when you take your grief and teach it to smile.

You are brave . . . when you overcome your fear and help others to do the same.

You are happy . . . when you see a flower and are thankful for the blessing.

You love . . . when your own pain does not blind you to the pain of others.

You are wise . . . when you know the limits of your wisdom.

You are true . . . when you admit there are times you fool yourself.

You are alive . . . when tomorrow's hope means more to you than yesterday's mistake.

You are growing . . . when you know what you are but not what you are becoming.

You are free . . . when you are in control of yourself but do not wish to control others.

You are honorable . . . when you find your honor is to honor others.

You are generous . . . when you can give as sweetly as you take.

You are humble . . . when you do not know how humble you are.

You are beautiful . . . when you don't need a mirror to tell you.

You are rich . . . when you never need more than you have.

\*\*\*\*\*\*\*\*\*\*\*\*\*\*\*\*\*\*\*\*\*\*\*\*\*\*\*\*\*\*\*\*\*\*\*\*\*\*\*\*\*\*\*\*\*\*\*\*\*\*\*\*

At the end of the day when we crawl into bed and all the lights go out, our thoughts will finally rise to the surface. Yes, we're a little bruised, slightly broken, and permanently scarred but we're still here aren't we? We're still fighting, we're still waking up every day to go through it all over again. This life may be hard as hell but it's still a gift and we all should get going to live every moment of it.

(Jerose Bautista)

A little faith will bring your soul to heaven, but a lot of faith will bring heaven to your soul.

(Martin Luther King)

Our greatness lays not so much in being able to remake the world as in being able to remake ourselves.

(Mahatma Gandhi)

Changing the way you feel is easy compared to running around trying to change the circumstances of the outside world. Change your feelings and the outside circumstances will change.

(Rhonda Byrne)

The most beautiful people we have known are those who have known defeat, known suffering, known struggle, known loss, and have found their way out of the depths. These persons have an appreciation, sensitivity, and an understanding of life that fills them with compassion, gentleness and a deep loving concern. Beautiful people do not just happen.

Believe in yourself and all that you are. Know that there is something inside you that is greater than any obstacle.

No one is useless in this world that lightens the burden of it for anyone else.

(Charles Dickens)

Change is hard. You fight to hold on and you fight to let go . . . in the end, we all know change is needed for you to grow. After all, The Caterpillar never knew it was going to be a Butterfly!

Choose your thoughts carefully. Keep what brings you peace, release what brings you suffering. And know that happiness is just a thought away!

Nothing continues except change; nothing remains the same, nor should it. Life is not a state of being, but a process of becoming. To go anywhere, we must leave where we are; to become anything else, we must stop being what we were . . .

(Jules Z. Willing)

Being brave is not just about rescuing someone from a burning building or fighting crime or Lassie saving Timmy from the well. It's also about being brave enough to get out of bed every single day and face your life with grace in spite of being out of work, in chronic pain or experiencing loss and grief . . .

**WHAT HAPPENS TO GOOD PEOPLE WHEN BAD THINGS HAPPEN TO THEM?**
**THEY BECOME BETTER PEOPLE!**

**\*\*\*\*\*\*\*\*\*\*\*\*\*\*\*\*\*\*\*\*\*\*\*\*\*\*\*\*\*\*\*\*\*\*\*\*\*\*\*\***

# Appendix Three

## Useful Resources List

*The following list is by no means exhaustive.*

*It is MY compilation of useful resources and I hope you may find some of these suggestions useful to your own personal growth (or they provide links to further valuable information).*
This list (services or people) is not endorsed by anyone, *and is based on a WHOLE person approach, which means that it includes websites, organisations, contacts and people*—some *of whom have helped me personally, not only through my experience with FMS, but also enhanced my personal growth, learning and knowledge.*

## Tracey Jane (Clinical Psychologist)

Team member at *Connected Self.* www.connected self.com.au/about-us/about-us

*Connected Self*-Connection Inspiration Innovation.

19 Portrush Road, Payneham
Telephone—08 8362 6610.

## Jacob Teitelbaum, M.D

Jacob Teitelbaum, MD, is a board certified internist and Medical Director of the national Fibromyalgia and Fatigue Centers and Chronicity. He is author of the popular free iPhone application "Cures A-Z," and author of the best-selling book From Fatigued to Fantastic! (Avery/Penguin Group), Pain Free 1-2-3 (McGraw-Hill), Three Steps to Happiness: Healing Through Joy (Deva Press 2003), Beat Sugar Addiction NOW! (Fairwinds Press, 2010), and his newest book Real Cause, Real Cure (Rodale Press, July 15, 2011).

Dr. Teitelbaum *knows CFS/fibromyalgia as an insider*— he contracted CFS when he was in medical school and had to drop out for a year to recover. In the ensuing 25 years, he has **dedicated his career to finding effective treatment.**

Website www.EndFatigue.com

Facebook page http://www.facebook.com/DrTeitelbaum

## *Finding Ur Wings* Facebook Page

For more information about Ros and/or to 'connect' with her please refer also to her website . . .

http://findingurwings.yolasite.com/

## *De-Stress and Be Happy* Facebook page

Kerry offers a wide range of services! Refer also to website for more information . . .

www.kerryheritage.com.au/

## Deirdre Rawlings—'Foods for Fibromyalgia'

Deirdre Rawlings is traditional naturopath, certified nutritionist, sports nutritionist, master herbalist, and certified health and wellness coach. She holds a PhD in holistic nutrition, a Master's in holistic nutrition, a master's in herbal medicine, and is board certified by the American Naturopathic Medical Certification Board, and Wellcoaches ®.

Deirdre's passion for holistic medicine was ignited by her *success in healing her own* chronic fatigue, food allergies, digestive issues, hormone imbalances, and adrenal deficiency. She combines almost two decades of experience in living vibrantly and sharing the latest scientific health principles and practices **to help people to experience the amazing healing powers of food and nutrition.**

Deirdre specializes in hormone and blood sugar balance, chronic fatigue, fibromyalgia, digestive problems, food allergies, hypertension, adrenal/ energy deficiency, cleansing and detoxification. She is the author of several books.

Websites:

www.FoodsForFibromyalgia.com

www.Nutri-Living.com

www.DASHDietFoods.com

## MARY SHOMON; THYROID PATIENT ADVOCATE

Mary Shomon is a patient advocate, writer, communicator, and hormone patient. She has transformed her own struggle with thyroid disease into an advocacy campaign on behalf of patients with *chronic diseases* such as **thyroid disease, autoimmune conditions, chronic fatigue, and others**.

http://www.thyroidcoaching.com/

http://www.thyroid-info.com/

http://thyroid.about.com/

## Sandra Cabot

Dr. Sandra Cabot, a medical doctor for over 30 years, is the author of 21 books on health, including the famous **Liver** Cleansing Diet book and other subjects including **hormone health**. www.sandracabot.com/

## Dr James Wilson

Dr James Wilson is very well known and well informed in regards to the important relationship between stress and **adrenal fatigue** and how these areas impact on our health. He is also the Author of *'Adrenal Fatigue: The 21st Century Stress Syndrome'* and formulator of Dr. Wilson's Original Formulations. Dr. Wilson's mission is to help create a healthier world, person by person. www.adrenalfatigue.org

(**Understanding adrenal function** is another important part of understanding FMS. If/when adrenal gland function reduces; every system and organ in your body may be affected. If a decrease in adrenal hormones is experienced, then your body will attempt to make up for this underactivity—but this further influences many systems, and may result in alterations at the biochemical and cellular levels. ADRENAL FATIGUE CAN RESULT IN DRAMATIC IMPACT(S) ON QUALITY OF LIFE.)

## OTHER RELEVANT AND USEFUL INFORMATION AND CONTACTS;

**www.centrelink.gov.au/internet/internet.nsf/ home/index.htm**

For Information on **eligibility** and *other relevant basic guidelines* regarding—Sickness benefits, Disability payment, Health Care card and other concessions, reduced capacity assessment etc.

**www.fibromyalgia-symptoms.org/fibromyalgia _naturopath.html**

Explanation of the use of **Naturopath's** in the treatment of fibromyalgia. Includes types of treatments (options) which may be used and how the treatment may help. Also explains what to expect from a Naturopath and tips on how to find a suitable Naturopath.

**www.racgp.org.au/factsheets**

Provides information for consumers regarding the **'GP Mental Health Care Plan'.** What it is, how you may benefit, using the plan, and how to access more information. (The Royal Australian College of General Practitioners).

**www.beyondblue.org.au**

The National **Depression** Initiative.

**www.actmindfully.com.au/mindfulness**

**Provides links to useful information about Mindfulness**. Includes information and explanations, and definitions of 'mindfulness'—example 'Awareness of present experience with acceptance'— Germer, Segal, Fulton. Mindfulness is about waking up, connecting with ourselves, and appreciating the fullness of each moment of life. A profound way to enhance psychological and emotional resilience, and to increase life satisfaction. Increasingly recognised as an effective way to increase fulfilment, reduce stress, raise self-awareness, enhance emotional intelligence, and undermine destructive emotive, cognitive, and behavioural processes. Mindfulness DOES NOT mean meditation.

**http://makingaustraliahappy.abc.net.au/mindfulness.php**

About mindfulness (**Dr Russ Harris)**.

**http://mindfulnesscentre.com/about-us.html**

Australian based, the Mindfulness Centre was launched in 2006. Head Office is based in Goodwood, South Australia. *'Offering tools to help people move beyond the depression, stress, overwhelm, self doubt, indecision and other challenging emotions that stress and trouble everybody'.*

www.arthritissa.org.au/aspx/fibromyalgia.aspx

**Supports People with Fibromyalgia in South Australia** via self management courses, regular newsletter, information/education sessions, a telephone advisory service as well as support groups.

www.bridgesandpathways.org.au/index.php

*'Beyond Chronic Illness'*—Bridges and Pathways Institute Inc., South Australia. Includes updates on research and service delivery model, links to self help/self management, Fibromyalgia Australia, networking, Multiple Chemical Sensitivities, Training and work pathways, Peer Workers, Chronic Pain Consumer Network.

www.sasma.org.au/links.html

*'South Australian Self Management Alliance'*, Empowering Consumers Through Collaboration.

www.painmanagement.org.au/self-help

Australian Pain Management Association (**Self Help**).

www.chronicillness.org.au/community.htm

**Chronic Illness Alliance**. Representing over 40 consumer and advocacy groups on matters of common concern. Includes a directory (links) of Chronic Illness Alliance Members' Websites.

**www.cfidsselfhelp.org/about-us/bruce-camp bell-bio**

**'Practical Tools for Managing Chronic Fatigue Syndrome and Fibromyalgia'**. Includes access to online self—management courses.

**www.health.gov.au/internet/main/publishing. nsf/Content/mbsprimarycare-chronic**

**MBS Primary Care Items**—'Chronic Disease Management (CDM) Medicare Items. Explains CDM items and Medicare Benefits Schedule for chronic/ complex care needs. Provides links, fact sheets, Questions and answers, links to other resources.

**www.healthinsite.gov.au/topics/Chronic_ Disease_Management**

**'Self Management of Chronic Diseases'**. Provides links to information on self management or self care for people with Chronic illnesses.

www.health.gov.au/internet/publications/
publishing.nsf/Content/mental

**'Prolonged Fatigue Syndromes',** Clinical guidelines explaining possible causes of 'prolonged fatigue', assessment (causes), investigations, treatment.

\*\* In addition to these reference points—there are also many links now available (online) that provide information on research outcomes and associated documents. However, as this book has been largely 'non clinically' based *I have chosen NOT to list and include information of this nature*—but encourage each individual to do their own research in this regard. \*\*

# Appendix Four

## Recommended Books

Aisbett, Bev. 2008. *'The Book of IT'*. Pymble NSW: HarperCollins.

Albom, Mitch. 2009. *'Have a Little faith'*. New York: Hyperion.

Albom, Mitch. 1997. *'Tuesdays With Morrie'*. New York: Doubleday.

Bailey, Sam. 2006. *'Head Over Heels'*. Sydney NSW: ABC Books.

Bottomley, David & Maulucci Rita. 2008. *'Stop Surviving—Live Your Life'*. Pyrmont NSW: Fairfax Media Publications Pty Ltd.

Cabot, Dr Sandra. 1997. *'Boost Your Energy'*. Paddington, NSW: WHAS.

Carl, Glenys. 2006. *'Hold My Hand—A Mothers Journey'*. London: Pan Books.

Carter, Abigail. 2009. *'The Alchemy of Loss—A young widows transformation'*. Sydney NSW: Hachette Aust.

Chamberlain, Yvonne. 2008. *'Why Me ? Kicking cancer and other life changing stuff'*. Vic: YC.

Cloud, Henry. 2006. *'Complete Guide to Boundaries'*. Sydney NSW: Strand.

Davies, Lisa. 2009. *'True Colours; Lauren Huxley and her family; From tragedy to triumph'*. Pymble NSW: HarperCollins.

Edwards, Gill. 2007. *'Life Is A Gift'*. London: Piatkus Books Ltd.

Fox, Michael J. 2009. *'Always Looking Up—the adventures of an incurable optimist'*. London: Ebury Press.

Fox, Michael J. 2002. *'Lucky Man'*. Milsons Point NSW: Bantam.

Gawler, Grace. 2008. *'Grace, Grit and Gratitude'*. Ocean Shores NSW: Grace Gawler.

Greive, Bradley T. 2004. *'The book for people who do too much'*. Aust: Random House.

Gyatso, Geshe Kelsang. 2005. *'How to Solve Our Human Problems'*. Ulverston, England: Tharpa Publications.

Harris, Dr Russ. 2007. *'The Happiness Trap'*. Wollombi, NSW: Exisle Publishing Limited.

Hassed, Craig. 2002. *'Know Thyself—The Stress Release Programme'*. Melbourne Vic: Michelle Anderson Publishing.

Hay, Louise. 1982. *'Heal Your Body'*. USA: Hay House, Inc.

Hay, Louise. 2007. *'The Present Moment; 365 daily Affirmations'*. California: Hay House, Inc.

Hay, Louise. 1994. *'Meditations To Heal Your Life'*. California: Hay House, Inc.

Hayes, Tania. 2008. *'Love Has No Limits'*. Chatswood, NSW: Mira Books.

Koenig, Cheryl. 2008. *'Paper Cranes ; A Mothers story of hope, courage and determination'*. Auckland: Hourglass.

LaRoche, Loretta. 2003. *'Life is Short . . . . Wear your party pants'*. Carlsbad California: Hay House, Inc.

Leigh, Wendy. 2009. *'Patrick Swayze—One Last Dance'*. New York: Simon Spotlight Entertainment.

Matthews, Andrew. 2005. *'Happiness Now'*. Trinity Beach QLD: Seashell Publishers.

McClarty, Gene. 2006. *'Live Life to the Full'*. Norwood South Australia: Peacock Publications.

Nicholas, Dr Michael., Molloy, Dr Allan., Tonkin, Lois. & Beeston, Lee. 2000.*'Manage Your Pain; Practical and positive ways of adapting to chronic pain'*. Sydney: ABC Books.

O'Brien, Chris. 2008. *'Never Say Die'*. Pymble NSW: HarperCollins Publishers.

Opie, Jenny. 2005. *'Simple Truths'*. South Australia: Axiom Publishing.

Pausch, Randy. 2008. *'The Last Lecture'*. Sydney NSW: Hachette Australia.

Scott, Sophie. 2010. *'Roadtesting Happiness; How to be happier (no matter what)'*. Pymble NSW: ABC Books.

Teitelbaum, Jacob. 2007. *'From Fatigued to Fantastic'*. New York: Penguin Group Inc.

Virtue, Doreen. 2007. *'Healing Words From the Angels'*. California: Hay House, Inc.